The Sick Doctor
by Dr. Gabrielle Koczab

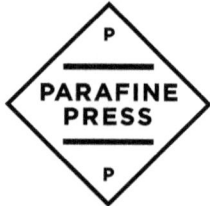

Parafine Press 3143 W.33rd Street, #6 Cleveland, Ohio 44109 www.parafinepress.com
Printed in the United States of America

Dedication

This autobiographical work is the diary I kept as I battled breast cancer. I have included my poetry as well. Writing has been therapeutic during this journey. This nonfiction work is dedicated to my son, Elliot, who came up with the title. I will never forget the day my five-year-old came to me and said, "Mommy, you should write a book. A grown-up book with bad words in it. And you can call it *The Sick Doctor*." I also dedicate this work to my husband, who showed up every day for this shitshow.

Preface

Before Elliot came to me with his book idea and title, I was already strongly considering writing a book. I was going to call it "The Red Brick Road." In the movie *The Wizard of Oz*, Dorothy must follow the yellow brick road full of twists and turns in order to find her way to the Emerald City, after the twister lands her in the middle of Munchkinland. It is a quest to find her way home. In the beginning, the yellow brick road is intertwined with the red brick road. The red brick road eventually trails off. But where does that red brick road go? It is a question without an answer. It reminds me of my life, which is filled with uncertainty. This is the journal I kept throughout my treatment. It is interspersed with the poems I wrote throughout my cancer journey. I have found writing poetry and journaling to be incredibly therapeutic. This journey is more of a rollercoaster ride with ups and downs on an uncharted path. It is also a story about the intertwining of the role of a physician with that of a patient.

Here I was: a busy working-doctor-mommy running a family medicine residency clinic. On most days, I was burning the candle at both ends. I was up by 4:30 a.m. every morning. I would walk the dog or work out at the gym before going to work. Then, I would work from about 7:00 a.m. until 5:00 or 5:30 p.m. Sometimes, I would have evening meetings and I wouldn't arrive home until 8:30 or 9:00 p.m. Then, suddenly, I was sidelined with invasive breast cancer at thirty-eight years old. This is a place I thought I would never be in my life. Moms are not supposed to get sick. Doctors are not supposed to get sick. People in their thirties and forties, the prime of their lives, are not supposed to get sick. Yet, here I am. Cancer, the dreaded "C" word, affects every hat I wear.

I can only describe the feeling like being swept to a foreign land. It is as terrifying as it was for Dorothy when she landed in a faraway place she had never seen before.

And you just want to click your heels together three times to suddenly wake up in your own home and go back to the way things used to be.

Chapter 1

"You just have to take it one 'are you fucking kidding me' at a time." –Unknown Author

April 8, 2019. "Katie, will you write me an order for a diagnostic mammogram?" I say to my nurse practitioner. Katie is more than just my employee; she is a friend. We have shared an office for the past two years. Serving as the medical director of our primary care practice, I am Katie's collaborating physician. We have grown close over a short period of time. When I met her, I felt I had already known her for years. She is one of the few people I've felt this about. Katie was the one who found my cancer after I confided in her that I was having sharp pains in my left breast, and that the tip of my left nipple was turning grayish in color. My gut feeling told me that I had stage 2 breast cancer.

Gut feelings are guardian angels. As a third-year medical student, I remember being on my inpatient Internal Medicine rotation taking care of a patient who was admitted for chest pain. His initial EKG (heart tracing) and blood levels for cardiac markers were negative in the emergency room for a myocardial infarction, or heart attack. He was admitted to the observation unit just to make sure a heart attack was not evolving. This patient of mine, "Joe," was a pleasant man who had been brushed off by the cardiology resident. I had a gut feeling about Joe that something was terribly wrong—although I didn't know exactly what it was. As a third-year medical student who had just started clinical rotations, I was not taken very seriously by the senior residents. I pleaded with the attending physician to order a spiral CT scan of his chest. A few hours later, my attending physician paged me to tell me, "Gabby, your patient has a dissecting aortic aneurysm and you probably just saved his life." That was over fourteen years ago, and I still remember that moment as if it was yesterday.

Now it was I who had this gut feeling about something very wrong in my own body. It was a Thursday and I figured the test would not take very long, so I made the short walk through the hospital from my office to the radiology department, and, shortly afterwards, I found myself in the land of unknowns. I was between patients when I went down for the mammogram. After it was over, I had a short conversation with the radiologist that I will never forget. The date was April 11, 2019. I was thirty-seven years old, about to turn thirty-eight the following week. Immediately after my mammogram pictures were taken, my coworker—the head radiologist—sat down with me. He told me, "It doesn't look good, Gabby. I am going to call Lisa on your behalf." Dr. Lisa Rock is a breast surgeon and she serves as the medical director of the breast center for our hospital system. I could recall scrubbing surgeries with her fourteen or fifteen years ago as a medical student. And here she was, about to become my doctor. I was terrified, but on some level it felt serendipitous.

On Friday, April 12, I arrived at the breast center as a terrified patient and not as a confident physician. I spent almost four hours there. First, I had an office visit with Dr. Rock followed by a breast ultrasound. They were able to visualize a mass to biopsy. The interventional radiologist performed an ultrasound-guided biopsy of five spots on my left breast. I cried throughout the entire thing. It was not physically painful, but, when I saw the ultrasound screen, I just knew. I am not a radiologist, nor do I have any formal training in ultrasound, but it was my gut feeling again. The nurse who was assisting her was trying to make me feel better by telling me about her personal experience with breast cancer. She also told me that there were many patients with much worse findings on imaging who had great outcomes. None of those statements provided any comfort. She offered me a small tube of lavender essential oil. I felt like a wreck. There was no fucking way that this octopus-shaped mass I was seeing on the screen was benign. April 12, 2019 was an emotional day. While waiting for the pathology results during the weekend, I could not empty my brain of invading thoughts about cancer. What type was it? What stage was it? My mind felt like the twister that took Dorothy away from the comfort of her home and transported her to a bizarre foreign territory.

Chapter 2

"Start with fear. Start with doubt. Start with shaking hands. Start with a numb brain. Start with bleeding back. Start with empty chest. Start with no light. Start with blinding glare. Start with trembling bones. Start with fog or start with night. Start with dawn or start with faint sight. But you my warrior princess, start you must." –Nivedita Lakhera

April 13, 2019. Reflecting back, I had a pretty good childhood. I grew up in the working-class neighborhood of East Detroit (now Eastpointe) in the eighties and nineties. I spent most days playing with the other kids in the neighborhood until the sun went down. We had a community park and pool nearby. Recalling these memories makes me smile. My younger brother, Ben, and I would travel around the neighborhood on our bikes and come in finally when the sun went down. I miss those summer days of being dirty and itchy from mosquito bites. Fast-forward to the summer of 2019: this summer was shaping up to be the worst summer of my life so far. I wish so badly that I could rewind time to these carefree days when the word "cancer" was not part of my vocabulary.

I had decided early on that I wanted to be a physician. When I was fourteen, I started volunteering at the largest hospital in Detroit. My friends and I would go there every Friday evening and some weekends here and there too. We would pass out cups of water, deliver flowers, and feed patients. I loved kids and babysat in my spare time. At this point in my life, I was determined to become a pediatrician. One of my favorite things to do was to visit the pediatric ward in the hospital while volunteering. I would scoop up little babies from their cribs and hold them, taking care not to disturb the IV tubing or wires that were attached to their tiny bodies. The nurses were amazed at the gift I possessed. The babies relaxed with me and I was able to handle their fragility with the ease of a seasoned pediatrics nurse.

From sixth grade on, I had basically committed to studying science and medicine and to becoming a doctor. If I made it through medical school, I would be the first in my family to hold a doctorate. My family was full of hardworking individuals but none had gone into medicine. No one in my immediate family even possessed an advanced degree. I did not have anyone to give me practical advice about how to succeed at this goal. I just figured it out on my own. In fact, I had several naysayers along the way. Their voices have stuck in my head to this day. Even my high school guidance counselor, who met with me in his office after I bombed my pre-ACT test, tried to talk me into an easier path and a different career choice. "Why don't you go to community college?" he said. That advice stayed in the back of my mind as I rocked my real ACTs the following year and earned a full-ride academic college scholarship.

After a wonderful four years of college in Cleveland, two hundred miles away from my family, I moved even further east. Erie, Pennsylvania was very different from Cleveland or Detroit. Erie was smaller and it was my perception that everyone seemed to know everyone else. Lake Erie College of Osteopathic Medicine accepted me as a medical student and I started there in late July 2003. My boyfriend (now husband) and I moved into a one-bedroom apartment near the lake. As an independent-study student, I spent the early part of the day studying and then I would meet up with a few friends to quiz each other before exams. Once I finished anatomy lab, I only had to be on campus one day per week. I graduated with honors on June 10, 2007, the first physician in my family. The challenges of medical school would pale in comparison to what I faced as a cancer patient.

Chapter 3

"These mountains that you are carrying, you were only supposed to climb." –Najwa Zebian

April 15, 2019. I just got off the phone with Dr. Rock. My table hasn't just turned; it has completely flipped upside down. One moment ago I was a physician, medical director, and division chair of family medicine. Now I am officially a breast cancer patient! Shocked and stunned, I pleaded with her to take me to surgery the next day and "get it out of there!" The pathology report read, "High grade DCIS, or ductal carcinoma in-situ." Since the cancer is confined to the milk duct, physicians refer to this as stage 0 breast cancer. Dr. Rock explained it didn't work that way. Yes, I needed a mastectomy but not tomorrow! I needed to do a breast MRI for them to evaluate the extent of the disease. After that, I needed to see the genetics counselor for special genetics testing due to my young age. Finally, I would need to see the plastic surgeon to discuss reconstruction options. Only five percent of breast cancer patients are under the age of forty. Why me and why now? And how in the hell do I concentrate on my own patients' health care needs when I have just been hit in the face with a cancer diagnosis?

As a teenager, I had read every one of Lurlene McDaniel's books. She writes young adult novels about young people facing a health crisis such as cancer or needing a heart transplant. I spent countless hours volunteering at the hospital in my teenage years. After that, I trained and worked as a primary care physician. During my first two years of medical school, I even volunteered at Shriner's Hospital and saw many children with severe orthopedic issues. In addition, my own mother has battled her own serious health issues. I thought I knew how these patients and parents of sick children felt, as I was a very empathetic and compassionate person. But nothing prepared me for the amount of fear and uncertainty that flooded me. It is, at times, too intense to describe in words. The panic attacks and nightmares that invaded my mind could be terrifying. One particular night, I dreamt of buying a plane ticket to Oregon and dying peacefully by legal-physician-assisted suicide. I woke up sweating and shaking a few times from these nightmares. I also had nightmares about living in denial and not showing up for surgery. The first days after hearing the "C word" were physically, emotionally, and mentally draining. I saw a therapist, and even he could not find any words to help me.

My list of worries went on and on and I had so many questions:

- Would my husband still want me without breasts?

- Would I bleed to death in surgery?

- Could the cancer itself spread and kill me?

- I have always been very independent, but would I be able to take care of myself after surgery?

- I have a husband and a small child that rely on me financially; would I be able to take care of my family?

- If I have to take a lot of time off work, what would I do with my student loans?

- How would I deal with my altered appearance after surgery? Would I feel ugly?

- How would I maintain privacy with patients?

- Would I have constant post-mastectomy pain after surgery?

- Would the medication give me bad side effects?

- Would I be able to cope emotionally?

- Would this scare friends and family members away or bring us closer?

- Would I be able to attend my brother's wedding in a few months?"

Only time would tell.

Ignore Your Suffering

You are a college senior about to take a big test,
You're running a fever and really need rest.
Your professor tells you to come back next week,
And sit for the exam when you are back at your peak.
In medical school, you have surgery your first year,
You only miss a few days not wanting to hurt your career.
Ignore your suffering ignore your pain.
Push through fever or with a throbbing brain.
Get back up and move forward whether you are ready or not.
Show up to work barely breathing or when your head is hot.

When you become the patient, it doesn't seem right.
You're supposed to be the doctor so you keep up the fight.
You're looked at as a hero when you work through the pain.
When you ignore your suffering, there is profit to gain.
If you are contagious, you can just wear a mask.
Ignore your suffering; there are just so many tasks:
Your patients, your residents are counting on you to be there,
Although the pain might be almost too much to bear.
Show up to work, ignore your suffering; they need you.
The agony you hide deep inside continues to brew.
Wheezing, coughing you feel like death.
It shouldn't be this hard to take a damn breath.

When your patients are sick you tell them to stay home from work,
But when you take your own advice you feel like a jerk.
Your broken bone will heal whether you are at work or home.
Draw strength from your pain, you think with a groan.
Ignore your suffering and just get through the day.
Tomorrow you will be better, you lie to yourself, and say
You have been knocked down many times before,
But keep picking yourself back up off of the floor.

Ignore your suffering ignore your pain
People are counting on you and there are bills to pay.

So you continue to push even though you need care.
You always give so much more than your share.
One day you will retire and maybe then you will rest.
Until then, ignore your pain and do more than your best!

Chapter 4

"I am no longer interested in becoming unbreakable. I am interested in shattering with grace and courage, and making art of all the broken pieces."—Nisha Moodley

April 16, 2019. Today is my thirty-eighth hbirthday. Celebration is the furthest thing from my mind. My staff tries to brighten my day with colorful balloons. This morning, instead of seeing patients, I am scheduled for my breast MRI. A slightly irritable nurse inserts my IV for the MRI dye that must be injected. I lie face down on this hard piece with cutouts for my breasts. The MRI technician asks me what kind of music I want to listen to. It doesn't matter; even with headphones on, it is impossible to hear the music. Noise coming from the machine and noise coming from inside my head keep me occupied. My chest wall is sore by the time the twenty-five-minute test is over. I feel so vulnerable and scared. I want to cry, but I hold back the tears. I do not feel like the confident physician that I am at all. I feel like a completely different person. As I get dressed and ready to leave, I notice something in the mirror of the changing room—a couple of hives on my neck. I try not to panic in the twelve-minute drive back to the house, even though my throat feels a little tight. Is it tightness from a worsening allergic reaction or anxiety? I cannot tell. The moment I walk in the door I take a swig of my child's liquid allergy medicine. Just in case.

April 17, 2019. Today I see the genetics counselor. So many people have asked me the following question: "Is breast cancer in your family?" Three out of four of my grandparents had cancer of varying types. My nana (maternal grandmother) had very early stage breast cancer in her sixties. I remember dyeing my hair pink and visiting her in the hospital. She had a unilateral mastectomy, but no radiation or chemotherapy. She lived twelve more years and then passed away from a health issue unrelated to her cancer. My papa (maternal grandfather) died of pancreatic cancer in his early sixties. He was like me in that he did not smoke or drink, he exercised, and ate pretty healthily. My grandfather on my father's side died of bone cancer. No one else in my family had been diagnosed with cancer at my age. Why me? I don't smoke, I don't drink, and I don't use drugs. I eat fairly healthy food and I exercise. For years, I have eaten tons of foods that are supposed to be "anti-cancer." Every morning I drink green tea, and every day I have some dark chocolate. I eat organic kale and I drink chlorophyll water, damn it! What a giant slap in the face cancer is.

The one month between diagnosis and mastectomy was painful. Not physically painful, but emotionally painful. I had an insanely hard time concentrating at work. I had to call a patient about her abnormal mammogram results, and, for the first time in my life, it felt strange. Very strange. I don't think the patient could tell I was shuddering knowing she would have to undergo a breast biopsy. Silently and desperately shouting into the universe with the hope that she would not get the same results as I did. I suspected that she was going to have the same kind of breast biopsy I just had just gone through the week before. After I hung up the phone with her, I checked my MRI results. The mass was 6.6 x 2.0 x 2.5 cm in the left breast. I looked at the images on the computer with Katie. There was no way that it was just confined to the duct. Half the breast was lighting up! But I took a breath and I held onto a shred of hope that it was not invasive. The lymph nodes appeared normal. I was looking for any silver lining in all of this.

At this point, I don't know how to answer the simple question, "How are you?" Everyone keeps asking. I am overwhelmed. It is hard to eat or sleep. It feels like drowning. A friend of mine said to me, "You are the last person on Earth I would ever imagine getting cancer. You eat vegetables! You drink green plant juice! You exercise! You don't drink pop!" I am trying very hard to shift my thinking from "why me," to "what is this trying to teach me?" And cancer class has just begun.

Chapter 5

"Being negative only makes the journey more difficult. You may have been given a cactus, but you don't have to sit on it!"—Unknown Author

April 20, 2019. Time is moving forward as it always does. I am scared shitless. I am trying to control the cancer and not have it control me. Today I purchased some mastectomy shirts that are soft oversized tops with snaps on the front and inside pockets for JP drains. After the surgeon removes your breasts, there is an empty space left that can collect fluid, so they insert these drains to suction it out. Gross. Before the big C, I had no idea mastectomy clothing even existed. Not only do mastectomy clothing and bras exist, but there are entire stores dedicated to selling these items. The lessons continue. My specialty is family medicine and osteopathic manipulation, not surgical. I vaguely remember my surgical rotations as a medical student and resident. I remember scrubbing in and learning the names of the instruments. Students are often relegated to holding retractors and occasionally suturing. Sometimes I took photos for the surgical team. In outpatient family medicine, the biggest "surgery" I would perform was a skin biopsy or mole removal, generally requiring no more than two sutures.

Everyone has been so kind to me, offering to put me in touch with their friends or family members who have had breast cancer. I am overwhelmed with the outpouring of support. I host Easter brunch at my house for my parents and my in-laws (my idea). My mom brings me a bright pink-red lipstick to wear on the day of the surgery, just like Geralyn Lucas—the author of "Why I Wore Lipstick to My Mastectomy." My current emotional state prevents me from remembering the content of the book. I am guessing Geralyn still wanted to feel pretty in a very ugly situation.

I am keeping busy at work taking care of my patients and teaching my residents. In between the usual work and home busyness, I am making lists of questions to ask the breast surgeon and the plastic surgeon. I have made lists of things I want to have during my medical leave, like my favorite Moroccan mint green tea and natural frankincense soap. Also, there are the lists of things that need to be completed, like my FMLA (Federal Family Medical Leave Act) and short-term disability forms, living will, and Health Care Power of Attorney. I marginally regret waiting until a serious disease occurred to do this. Here is some free advice: get your legal documents in order now. I bought life insurance over ten years ago, shortly after I tied the knot, but I never did complete my living will.

Chapter 6

"Wonder Woman is not a fictional character, but a mindset."—Unknown Author

April 22, 2019. Today I went in for an acupuncture treatment and I feel more relaxed. I called my student loan company and asked about the penalty-free cancer deferment bill that passed recently (House Bill 6157). The woman said the Department of Education is "working on it," but the forms have not yet been published or released. She tells me that, for now, they can put me into an administrative forbearance that does accumulate interest while we wait for the paperwork to be released. How defeating! I have paid my student loans on time every month for over ten years, and this feels like a punch in the gut. For a moment, it seemed a bit like I was being punished for being sick.

I cannot complain too much at the moment, as I feel grateful to have short-term disability pay through work. In addition, I purchased a separate long-term disability insurance policy as a medical student. I never thought I would have to use it. Cancer was not in my life plan. It was supposed to be one of those things that happened to other people, not to me. I am thankful that it is highly unlikely I will be among the forty-two percent of cancer patients that exhaust all of their savings in two years. Here is another tip: live below your means! Let me say that again: live below your means! I am not a financial expert like Suze Orman, but a Honda gets you just as far as a Mercedes. A purse from Target carries as much junk as a designer handbag. I am glad I made this decision to purchase long-term disability (LTD) insurance when I was in my twenties. Back then, I was young and healthy and it was cheap. As it turns out, this LTD insurance policy was worth the $680-per-year premiums I paid. I was not one that had to exhaust my savings, or tap into my 401(k), or beg for money online. My heart breaks for every single person who has to do this. Talk about being punished for being sick. The word "unfair" does not seem strong enough to describe it.

Chapter 7

"Perhaps the reason you are drawn to the flowers is not only because of their outer beauty, but because they remind you beautiful things will bloom after the longest seasons of waiting."
—Morgan Harper Nichols

April 23, 2019. I saw the plastic surgeon this morning. Both the nurse and the surgeon could not have been nicer to me. My one wish in life is that every physician would have the perfect balance of medical knowledge and a good bedside manner. I aim to be that way. As I was taken from the waiting room to the patient room, I passed a wall holding numerous brochures. I am overly sensitive right now and I become upset just thinking about it. The brochures were for liposuction, face-lifts, and "mommy makeovers." (Yes, there was an actual brochure called "Mommy Makeover.") Don't get me wrong. I understand that some people have deformities and need plastic surgery. But "mommy makeover?" The term implies that all moms are ugly and need surgery to look better. This made me feel nauseated and icky internally. While I have never been the first to sign up for a painful and dangerous surgery to change my appearance, I understand that everyone in the world has different priorities. People like myself are just here to see what the options are to look "normal" after cancer surgery. Despite the doctors' amazing bedside manner, I can still see the brochures in my mind. Next person to say, "Oh! You get a free boob job!" gets punched in the face. I do not want to be here!

In addition, I had to be measured and photographed in a very bright room, while I was completely naked. I can only describe the experience as humiliating. I am not sure I would even go through with reconstruction surgery. I am frightened to get implants due to the risks—silicone migrating or causing biofilm illness, sepsis (a bacterial blood stream infection), or breast-associated lymphomas. The only other option then would be a TRAM or DIEP procedure, in which they use your own fat or muscle from your abdomen to rebuild breast tissue. The plastic surgeon explained to me that the DIEP flap reconstruction is a major twelve-to-fourteen-hour surgery with a five-day hospital stay, up to six surgical drains and an eight-week recovery. I ask, "Can the DIEP reconstruction be performed at the same time as the mastectomy." No. If you end up needing radiation postoperatively, the radiation can ruin the tissue flap. Damn it.

Prosthetic breasts look like my main option at the moment. If I do not end up getting radiation, I cannot wrap my head around taking eight weeks off in the same calendar year. I will be taking six weeks off after the bilateral mastectomy. My head is spinning with all this information. There are so many decisions to be made. Cancer sucks. Why couldn't this have happened when I am in my sixties or seventies, financially set, and ready to retire anyway? End rant. Now that I have that out of my system, I am off to chuck axes with my family medicine residents. God, I love them! If you are reading this and you ever get dealt a bad hand in life, go axe throwing. It is a blast and a majorly cathartic activity. Honestly, this was one of the best evenings of my life. *I need to carve out time for more fun in my life*, I think to myself.

Chapter 8

"The strength you have comes from your head and your heart. You won't know how strong you are until you are asked to fight."—Ruth D'Hennin

April 24, 2019. The cancer itself is the least of my worries at this time. Right now it's the STRESS of all the appointments. And the STRESS of all the testing. And the STRESS of all the waiting. And the STRESS of missing work now and in the near future. And the STRESS about who will take care of my patients. And there's the STRESS of the finances. The STRESS of all of the "what ifs." And the STRESS of knowing I am going to have to depend on my family and friends. I am the one who always takes care of everyone else, not the other way around. Anyways, it is the STRESS that is just KILLING ME! Sorry, not sorry, I just had to scream it. As of today, I STILL don't have my exact mastectomy date, and it is freaking me out when I see words like "high grade" and "biopsy proven malignancy" on my medical reports. Despite all of this, I am still showing up to work every day. Life is tough, but so am I! The hardest part now is concentrating at work. How am I supposed to be compassionate and understanding with a patient who has the sniffles when I just got diagnosed with cancer? Concentrating on anything but the big C is just beyond difficult.

April 25, 2019. Dr. Rock called me today and we have set a surgery date. That date is May 15. I will stay in the hospital overnight. She has confirmed that she will do the bilateral mastectomy and the sentinel lymph node biopsy to see if there are any cancer cells in the nodes. Then, she wants the plastic surgeon to put in tissue expanders at the same time under the muscle in preparation for future reconstructive surgery. Reconstruction using my own tissue (DIEP) can be done at a later time. That is the surgery in which they perform a "tummy tuck" and use your own belly fat to rebuild your breasts. Both Dr. Rock and the plastic surgeon rave about how I am the perfect candidate for the DIEP flap reconstruction surgery because I am young, healthy, a non-smoker, not diabetic, and not too skinny, nor too fat. Apparently, not every patient meets these strict criteria. It is a lot to wrap my head around. Tissue expanders are similar to implants in my mind, and thoughts of sepsis or other complications start to invade my mind. Today I do not have to make this difficult decision and I am grateful for that. One day at a time.

April 26, 2019. My emotions are more down than up today, but I did get to the gym this morning for a workout, and then I went to Elliot's school. His pre-kindergarten class was putting on a play. Afterwards, we had breakfast at his school cafeteria. It was a lovely morning and it took my mind off some scary thoughts for a while. Honestly, how can you think about anything bad when your five-year-old son is a squirrel in a pre-K school play? But to be honest, for most of the time, my head is filled with anxiety, fear, anger, and rage.

I have to get this off my chest (no pun intended)! It is not helpful for anyone to tell me how to feel or what attitude to have. All feelings are valid when you have been diagnosed with fucking cancer! Hearing "Don't be angry!" or "Drop the attitude!" are not helpful remarks to someone who is pre-grieving the loss of her breasts, a part of her body, and her identity as a woman. Careless words can cause harm. Feelings are feelings, and you cannot just flick a switch and change them. It is near impossible. I am going through all of the Kubler-Ross stages of grief at once. From moment to moment I could feel anger, denial, bargaining, or intense sadness. Maybe one day I will make it to acceptance. The grieving process is not linear or easily controllable. Stress relief may come with acupuncture and meditation, but feelings cannot be erased like a chalkboard. Some days I wish feelings were like a light switch, and I could just turn them off. I've been dealt a really difficult hand here; I just need to have my emotions validated. I had a panic attack about the surgery date after I hung up the phone call with my surgeon, because it makes everything more real.

On a positive note, I am going to post some affirmations to try to keep my head from going to dark, scary places. Here goes: Today I am in charge. I am peaceful and present. I am strong and brave. In addition, I want to thank all of my friends and family for their concern, support, and help during this time. For those loved ones who want to know what they can do:

- Send handwritten cards or letters of encouragement.
- Send a text with a funny joke or meme.
- Send uplifting songs or titles of feel good or funny movies.

Chapter 9

"Some days I am a goddess. Some days I am wild child. And some days I am a fragile mess. Most days a bit of all three. But every day, I am here, trying."—S.C. Lourie

April 26, 2019. I was summoned for jury duty for May 22 (post-op day 6). Do I:

1. Show up a hot mess with drains coming out of me and scare everybody away? Or do I:

2. Get a doctor's note? (Rhetorical question).

Spoiler alert—I got a doctor's note. I do feel somewhat guilty about not going to jury duty. I was summoned once many years ago when I was a medical student and I told them I could not miss medical school. I asked them to contact me after June 30, 2010, my last day of residency. Ironically, they waited until I have a mastectomy planned to summon me. I understand the selection process is random, but still!

April 27, 2019. Today was a great day. Elliot and I played superheroes and threw a softball around the house. He was Captain America and I was the Black Widow. If I could only draw up the mental and physical toughness of a superhero right now to get me through cancer, it would be great. My husband and I went out on a date night. We had a great meal and saw *A Bronx Tale* down in Cleveland's Playhouse Square. What an amazing Broadway play! Here is an interesting fact—Chazz Palminteri, the main character of the play, was born on May 15, my surgery date. He grew up in a blue-collar family, just as I did, and he became famous. I doubt I will ever be as famous as him, but one can dream.

April 29, 2019. I have been busy over the last few days with organizing things. I met with an attorney who came by our house to help me prepare my legal documents (living will, health care power of attorney, guardianship paperwork, etc.) Here is a tip: if you do this at a younger age (i.e. in your twenties), it costs less. As I mentioned before, Marty and I bought life insurance shortly after we were married at age twenty-seven, but we never did our wills. My family can haggle over my possessions when I am gone—they are just things. I also filed for short-term disability through work and faxed in my medical excuse for jury duty.

Only fifteen days until surgery. I have found peace and comfort in an online private support group for women physicians with cancer. It is bittersweet that this group exists and there are several hundred women physicians in it. Some of them are survivors, some are cancer "lifers" who have metastatic disease, and some are early in their diagnosis like myself. Their diagnoses range from thyroid to breast to colon to malignant melanoma. Each one is a gem, unique and precious. I am so grateful for this group of women.

Life is a test and it tests you on every single level—emotionally, physically, spiritually, and financially. It tests your marriage and every single relationship. I am a wife, a mother, a doctor, a sister, and a friend. Cancer has put every single one of those roles to the test. A colleague gave me some great advice recently. She said to me, "Take control and realize that you are the one in charge. You are the one who will make decisions about your treatment." That phrase made me feel so empowered. Furthermore, getting my disability and living will paperwork in place well before surgery has reduced my anxiety even more.

Chapter 10

"The truth will set you free, but first it will piss you off."—Gloria Steinem

April 30, 2019. The genetics counselor called me today with my results. I do, in fact, have a genetic mutation that increases the lifetime risk of breast cancer to thirty-three to fifty-eight percent. It is the PALB2 gene and it is a cousin of BRCA 2, a gene that increases the risk of ovarian and breast cancer. PALB2 gene mutations are also associated with a possible increased risk of ovarian cancer and pancreatic cancer. Once I reach forty, I will qualify for pancreatic cancer screenings with this gene mutation. For once, my life journey makes some sense. For years I had a healthy lifestyle and I could not conceive a child. All of my infertility testing was normal and my husband's sperm count was in the range to be able to conceive naturally. We tried to have a child for five years, and for over two years I cleaned up my diet even more, had infertility acupuncture and I ingested Chinese herbal supplements from a physician certified to prescribe them. It was all for a reason—I would have been responsible for giving my natural-born child a difficult decision in the roulette of life. The child would have had to potentially opt for a prophylactic mastectomy by age thirty. This is a point of deep reflection. The universe has a way of working everything out in the end. If it's not working out, it's not the end. (Stole that one from the *Exotic Marigold Hotel* movie, but I love it!)

How do I have a five-year-old named Elliot if I did not conceive? Elliot grew in my heart, not my uterus. That is, he is adopted. After trying to conceive for about five years, Marty and I decided to pursue adoption. We selected a small private agency. The adoption process was an extremely difficult journey. We had an adoption fall through a few months before Elliot was born. Through a legal loophole, the birth mom was able to reclaim her baby eight days after he was born. The baby was born prematurely and he was still in the NICU, but for eight days I held him, rocked him, fed him, dressed him and read to him. We had bonded and I was his mother. When the adoption fell through, I did not think I could survive such pain. I think about him frequently and I hope he is thriving. Another life test.

My Path is My Path

I entered medical school in 2003,
A young bright healer, yes that's me,
Ready to tackle any challenge ahead.
Why didn't they warn me? No one said—
You will face attending physicians that will drag you down,
You will have so much on your plate that you'll want to drown,
You will hold the hands of people dying,
So sleep deprived you will feel like flying
Far away from the hospital call room,
Awakened by a code blue, the impending doom.
Then finally you graduate a real doc,
And here you still work around the clock.

One day you decide it's time for a baby.
Can't get pregnant, is it because work is crazy?
Is it too much stress? Is it the candy I ate?
The years pass by, is it getting too late?
Friends and family constantly ask me when.
Could the infertility be from the lack of zen?
So I go to yoga, run, sleep, and pray,
See my acupuncturist almost every day.
My path is my path with obstacles I face,
Some days my heart isn't always in the right place.

Five years pass by, I feel so empty inside.
Still no baby, my sadness I hide.
I go to work and see pregnant girls in despair,
Counseling them with compassionate care.
It is so difficult and sometimes I feel fake.
Life can be so painful, how much more can I take?
I apply for adoption, which seems like a good way
To finally have a little one and make my day.
So I go to the bank, take out a loan,
Jump through the hoops, wait by the phone.

The first match we get falls through really fast.
That child will not be ours, more days pass.
Finally a match that seems solid, we meet
A young couple who already has a baby to feed.
The baby is born premature, small but sweet.
We give him a name, come to the NICU to meet.
For eight days I held him, read to him and sang,
Not knowing on day eight that I'd feel so much pain.
As the adoption fell through, I fell to my knees and cried.
That day at the hospital, a part of me died.

The following week I returned to work and moved on,
Seeing my patients like I have done all along,
Running a lot to manage my stress.
Some days felt easy, some felt like a test.
Then in August of 2013,
I tripped and fell running; embarrassed by the scene,
I stood up and walked the five blocks back.
Bad pain in my left shoulder, I knew the bone cracked.
2013 was one hell of a year.
After all that I went through I am amazed I'm still here.

Then two days after running a half marathon race,
I received a phone call that lit up my face.
"You have a son," she said on my voicemail,
"He is 7 pounds 4 ounces, healthy and stable."
From that day on, I got to be a mamma,
But knowing my life there's got to be drama.
There was a bad ice storm our very first night,
We had to evacuate, I packed the diaper bag tight.
My path is my path and this is another bump in the road,
Sometimes I feel like I am carrying the heaviest load.

Another rough week September 2018,
Another time when my path was filled with weeds,
A patient of mine I had known for years died.
When I got the message, I sat down and cried.

Feeling sad and defeated, did I miss something? Drugs?
I had seen her the week prior and gave her a hug.
The same day a friend who is dear to my heart
Called me with news that hit me like a dart.
The baby girl inside her that she wanted so much,
Had gone with the angels never to be touched.

Some days my heart feels heavy, it's true.
Bad days are inevitable but good days are too.
Some days my path is full of thorns and branches, so thick.
The stress is so great I can feel physically sick.
I have quite a few scars, no doubt, but it is alright,
Scar tissue is stronger than regular and tight.
Life is for the living and so I will go and live it,
Working hard, playing hard, challenges you get it?
My path is my path and I will create it, not follow.
My emotions I carry them today and tomorrow.
As life gives me a test, I will try to embrace it,
And no matter the weather, I know I can face it!

Chapter 11

"You're only human, you don't have to have it together every moment of every day."
—Anne Hathaway

May 2, 2019. I saw both the breast surgeon and the plastic surgeon again this week. I have decided against any implants or tissue expanders due to the risks I have previously mentioned. I am feeling good about my decision and both doctors' acceptance of my choices. It seemed to me that they were initially pushing me to do the tissue expanders and then get the implants, but this is no longer the case. I can always return for a delayed breast reconstruction in the future, even if I am flat and fabulous. It is too overwhelming to me to think of doing multiple surgeries and exchanging tissue expanders for implants. I want to stay in control if, when, and where reconstructive surgery occurs. For now, I am controlling what I can control and I am staying relaxed with the help of acupuncture and guided meditation. My mind is still unfocused at times. I forgot about a meeting last night, which is not like me. I did not become the Division Chair of Family Medicine of my hospital at age thirty-six for no reason. I am lucky to have great colleagues who have had to cover for me during this time. I am feeling grateful at the moment. Thirteen days and counting until I will have the surgery.

May 3, 2019. I did not sleep well last night. I had a nightmare that seemed so real. I woke up shaky and sweaty. In my nightmare, I had uncontrollable pain and bleeding after the surgery. When I finally fell back asleep, Elliot woke me up at 11:30 p.m. and again at 2:30 a.m. because, "he loves me and misses me and wants to be by me." His words. Sleep regression doesn't just happen with babies and toddlers apparently. I try to remind myself they are only little once.

Eleven days and counting until surgery and six more work days. I made my appointment for my mastectomy post-op bra fitting for next week. My husband pointed out that the mastectomy store is no Victoria's Secret. If anyone who works for Victoria's Secret is reading this, please consider adding mastectomy bras to your inventory. On a positive note, the lady on the phone was genuinely nice and helpful. It makes me wonder how I am going to feel when I come out of surgery. Will I feel relieved that the cancer is gone from my body? Or will I be horrified when looking at my body? All I know is that it is probably going to be the biggest emotional and physical roller coaster of my life.

Chapter 12

"Life has a way of testing a person's will, either by having nothing happen at all, or having everything happen all at once."—Paulo Coelho

May 4, 2019. May the Fourth be with everyone today! This morning I went to see my allergist to figure out what I need to do in the future for my weird MRI dye allergy. Then I took advantage of a free massage at The Gathering Place, a place of support for patients and their families with cancer. The Gathering Place is amazing. They have support groups, a library, a wig salon, exercise classes, art therapy, and more. They have free Reiki and massage for cancer patients as well. And the more amazing thing is that it is funded solely through donations. Today my massage therapist asked me if I had any hobbies. Other than walking, running, playing with my kid, and occasionally reading books, not really, I tell her. I am too busy for hobbies. I am open to suggestions at this point, so I ask my family and friends for recommendations. Within a short period of time, I find myself with adult coloring books, novels, a puzzle, and a word game app for my cell phone.

May 5, 2019. Marty and I have a Sunday date night this weekend, instead of Saturday. We are down in the Cleveland Flats for dinner and a Leon Bridges concert. The weather is a tad chilly but almost perfect for an outdoor concert. Only ten more days until surgery, and I am determined to get out of the house as many times as possible until then. I have a great ambition in life: to die of exhaustion rather than boredom. I guess I just like to stay busy!

May 7, 2019. As the surgery date edges closer, I find myself feeling less peaceful and more anxious. There is no denying the rising fear inside of me. I don't want to be a patient. It is unnatural to me, the doctor. I am the one who always takes care of everyone else. I am not supposed to be a patient. There, I said it: I am afraid of having a bilateral mastectomy. I am even afraid of the words. I am afraid of how I will look the first time I see my warped body in the mirror. I am afraid of never being able to go to the gym again and change my clothes in the locker room. I am afraid the doctors will find more cancer in my lymph nodes. I am afraid of the pain that I am certain will come. I am afraid of reading my pathology report. I am afraid of the possibility of chemo or radiation. I am afraid of the possibility of losing my hair and feeling sick. I am afraid of being treated differently by everyone around me. I am afraid I will not just cry, but that I will sob for days. Sometimes, I feel like I won't even be able to walk into the hospital the day of my surgery. I am afraid I will freeze up and not be able to speak. My husband, family, and friends all try to reassure me, but I am still very afraid. More like terrified.

I am afraid of drain tubes, these plastic foreign objects inside my body meant to drain out the blood and fluid. My blood. The blood that should be inside of my body. I am afraid of scars. I am afraid I will not feel like a woman anymore once my breasts are amputated. A double mastectomy is so permanent. I am also afraid that my husband will see me as less desirable, as ugly. I am afraid he won't love me anymore, no matter how many times he tries to reassure me that he will. I am afraid of being weak and not being able to care for myself. Will I be able to take a shower and wash my hair? I have always been very strong, and it makes me feel vulnerable to admit all of this. I was never this afraid before. But if my journey can help me help others, it is all worth it. Seven-and-a-half days to go.

Chapter 13

"She will rise. With a spine of steel, and a roar like thunder, she will rise."—Nicole Lyons

May 8, 2019. Six days until surgery. I am fighting a little cold, so I contacted my surgeon to see if it would affect the procedure. She said as long as there is no fever or serious infection, everything will proceed as planned. Elliot is also under the weather. This is horrible timing! I cannot believe I have only three more work days left. I have not really told any of my patients why I am taking a leave of absence. I already feel scared and vulnerable enough; I am just not ready for all the pity looks and all the questions that will ensue. Overall, my patients have been lovely and respectful. I inwardly cringe when they tell me, with a big smile, to enjoy my time off. They probably think I am going on a vacation. I could use a vacation right now. Although Marty would say that I am a bad traveler, I do like to explore new places. I love eating at new and innovative restaurants, going to museums, watching shows, and shopping. We were married in Las Vegas and we have been there four times. Once I am done with all this cancer bullshit, I am taking a FUCK CANCER vacation!

May 10, 2019. I have only one day left of work. I am feeling bittersweet about things. I am in the process of changing roles at work. I practiced Family Medicine and Osteopathic Manipulation (OMT) for nine years, four of them in a family medicine residency clinic I started from scratch. The clinic was my baby. I started with a tiny office with just two staff members, a couple of residents, and three exam rooms. I did not even have an office and had to chart at the front desk. Now this practice has grown and expanded to a space with twelve exam rooms, six staff members, three providers, and six residents. It was stressful and hard work, but I am proud of it. I will miss everyone there so much. I am changing lanes from primary care to a new position in Integrative Medicine and OMT. I have always loved the patients that were considered "difficult" by other doctors. It is rewarding to me to uncover the root cause of the problem instead of covering up symptoms of fibromyalgia or chronic fatigue syndrome with medicine. Many times, I have found that there is an underlying cause such as nutritional deficiencies, undiagnosed food sensitivity, or even an undiagnosed tick-borne illness (Lyme disease, for example).

In other news, I went to acupuncture yesterday and then went to the mastectomy supply store to get some things. Who knew that there are at least a dozen different prosthetics to pick from? It was overwhelming to say the least. I continue to learn so much throughout this journey. As you might imagine, I am a little bit tired on every level right now—emotionally, physically, and spiritually. However, I will try to take the advice of Banksy, who said, "When you get tired, learn to rest, not quit!"

Chapter 14

"And just as the Phoenix rose from the ashes, she too will rise. Returning from the flames clothed in nothing but her strength, more beautiful than ever before."—Shannen Heartz

May 11, 2019. I am hanging out in downtown Cleveland today with my husband and son. We saw *Wild Kratts Live 2.0*, went to the coffee shop, the Cleveland Public Library, and then we had dinner at the House of Blues. Marty introduced Elliot to *The Blues Brothers* movie recently, and Elliot wore a black suit and fedora just like Jake and Elwood. The hostess at the House of Blues wanted to take his photo for the website so badly but Elliot refused. Even more, all of the concert-goers that evening pointed out how cool he looked. This has been a great day and another good distraction from my upcoming surgery in just four days.

May 12, 2019. Today I honor my journey to motherhood. It was a rough journey. Some days I did not think I would be able to make it through. At age twenty-seven, shortly after we got married, I was certain we would have a baby within a year or two. After two years of trying, we underwent infertility testing. Marty and I were told that we fell into the "unexplained infertility" category. Nothing seemed to be wrong with either of us. I went to acupuncture, cleaned up my diet, took herbal remedies, and exercised. I got my weight down. I prayed. Still, nothing happened. We decided against in vitro fertilization for various reasons before starting down the road to adoption. My heart felt like it was ripped in half the day we lost the first baby. I was so thankful the day Elliot came into our lives. I think about his birth mom often. She wanted a closed adoption, so we don't know anything about her, but I am incredibly amazed by and proud of any woman who can put her child's needs ahead of her own. Elliot even looks like Marty and I. People have a hard time believing he is not our biological kid. Like any child, there are times he makes me smile. Then, there are those moments when he makes me want to rip my hair out. However, without these struggles, I would have never found my strength. I wish I could find it now.

Reflecting on my story helps me gather my needed strength. I have survived hard times before. I need all the strength I can muster to get through my surgery in three days and through whatever else may lie ahead. I know my body will look very different in the mirror next week, but, as long as I still cast a shadow on the ground, I know that my presence and impact on the world is not over. Being a doctor and a mom is a struggle in itself, and, when you add cancer, it feels like the heaviest of burdens. Happy Mother's Day!

Chapter 15

"You wake up every morning fighting the same demons that left you so tired the night before and that, my love, is bravery."—Unknown Author

May 13, 2019. Today was my last day of patients for a while. For the most part, work was a great distraction from my own struggles. Work gave me a sense of purpose and a reminder of why I was put on this earth. Getting to know my patients and healing them is one of my greatest accomplishments. As I gently work on their bodies to treat their physical pain, I learn about them. They vary in ages from babies to geriatrics. Some are rich, some are middle class, and some are poor, but each one is a human being deserving of care in their time of need.

I am not going to lie—in the four weeks between biopsy-proven breast cancer and the surgery to treat it, some days were harder than others. What got me through it were my awesome patients, wonderfully supportive coworkers and residents. I mean, what other group of residents takes their attending physician to throw axes!

I have learned a tiny bit of how to let go of guilt, but it is still a work in progress. I am not perfect and I never will be, but, after the cancer diagnosis slapped me in the face, I had to cancel patients' appointments several times for my own appointments. Because I used to feel so guilty about doing this in the past, I would squeeze in patients whenever I could to make up the time. I would squeeze them in at 7:30 a.m. before clinic started, or at the end of the day. I would use my designated "administrative time" to squeeze in patients all the time. How I ever got my PowerPoint presentations done in time for my lectures to my students and residents was nothing short of a miracle. This time, though, I put my foot down. My own needs have to come first! It took over ten years and a life-changing event for me to put myself first, but I am moving forward in the classroom of life. Tomorrow I will be cleaning out my office, finishing up paperwork, and going to a final acupuncture session and some art therapy in my last day before surgery.

May 14, 2019. I went to The Gathering Place with Elliot today. The Gathering Place is a local center that provides cancer patients and their families with support. Before cancer, I did not know such a place existed so close to my home. Elliot and I drew pictures with one of the staff members there and spent time in the gardens outside as well. It was a beautiful sunny day. Surgery is only about twelve hours away now. I feel like I am somewhat at peace with things. I am overwhelmed with gratitude by the number of phone calls, text messages, and hugs today. I know that I am being transformed by this journey and just as Zig Ziglar states, *"Difficult roads can lead to amazing destinations."* One bad chapter in life does not mean my book is over, even though I sometimes feel I cannot turn one more page.

Chapter 16

"The wound is where the light enters you."—Rumi

May 15, 2019. Today is Surgery Day. My best friend, Heidi, drove in from Detroit to be with my husband and me. Heidi and I have known each other since second grade. We were in many of the same classes from second grade through sixth grade. She moved to a different city just prior to seventh grade, and, although some may have drifted apart after this, we grew closer. Maybe it's because the summer before eighth grade, Heidi broke her leg and I broke my arm. We were both in casts because she fell off of a rock playing mini-golf and I fell off of the slide at the playground. This was the last summer I can remember when I had to miss out on life events because of my health. It was twenty-five years ago. I could not swim with the cast on, and it was devastating to the twelve-year-old me.

Heidi and I remained close all throughout college. We visited seach other at our respective colleges, since our breaks were at different times. She attended college two hours north of Detroit and I attended college five hours south in Cleveland. Our paths were very different—I studied pre-medical sciences and she studied English and Communications. Our careers are just as opposite—Heidi owns a travel agency and I am a physician. Our tastes in music and food are also different. Hey, you know what they say: opposites attract. There is one thing that we do have in common though; we love shopping.

This day will live in my memory forever. Here I was, sitting on the hospital bed in the pre-op area of the hospital. Marty and Heidi were next to me. The anesthesiologist, one of my colleagues, was there to do his history and physical. There is something comforting, yet odd at the same time, when one of your colleagues is going to be putting you to sleep. Then Dr. Rock came in and shoved two long syringes into my left breast. These syringes were filled with the radioactive dye that would be taken up by the lymph nodes and "light up" if there was cancer in them. Weirdly, I wasn't that anxious. It must have been the midazolam they injected into my IV—a mild tranquilizer. I cannot recollect what happened from the moment I said good-bye to Marty and Heidi to the time I woke up in recovery.

Surprisingly, my chest didn't hurt that much when I woke up in the recovery area. The thing that bothered me the most was that my right hand was all tingly and numb. The numbness lasted for over a day. I started to panic about the fact that my hand could never regain feeling, which meant I wouldn't be able to perform manipulations on patients anymore. With all of the medications I was given, I was probably not thinking straight. In addition, my blood sugar was low after surgery and because of not eating anything for thirty-six hours. My nurse gave me IV fluids, which contained sugar, and she let me eat a sandwich. I had made it through the surgery. I was told my sentinel nodes were normal and I was so relieved. Dr. Rock sent my breast tissue and two nodes from the left breast to breast pathology. Just in case.

Chapter 17

"Never be ashamed of a scar. It simply means that you were stronger than whatever tried to hurt you."—Unknown Author

May 16, 2019. From my hospital bed, I can see out the window. The sun is shining and it looks like a beautiful spring day. My surgeon came to see me early this morning. I caught a glimpse of my chest when she unfastened my post-op bra to check my incisions. I did not scream or cry. I had a sense of calmness and I was reassured that the cancer was out of me. I kept peppermint essential oil at my bedside to help with the nausea, a side effect of the pain medication. Without breasts, I couldn't have breast cancer anymore. So I thought. I still have to wait on the final pathology for staging and treatment purposes. I was discharged home in the afternoon. My post-op instructions state to wait two days to shower. I was looking forward to my seeing my own furniture and the lack of beeping IV machines. I was looking forward to being in my own bed and eating my own food. But I was freaked out by having to empty my drains three times daily. These were shoved into my chest and filled up with bloody fluid. My chief resident came to my house for my first drain emptying experience. After that, I figured it out. Yes, I am a doctor but it had been over a decade since I had to care for surgical patients with drains.

May 17, 2019. Today is post-op day two. A friend of mine, who worked on inpatient oncology at the Cleveland Clinic, came over to help me shower and rebandage my drains. One of my old high school friends had sent me a recovery pouch. This life-changing recovery pouch is a mesh pouch that hangs around your neck to hold your drains while you shower. The simplest little things in life can make all the difference. The shower wore me out and I had to take two naps afterwards. I had never been happier to sleep in my own bed. My friends and family members sent us plenty of food, including my favorite—tacos and guacamole.

May 18, 2019. I am feeling a little bit stronger today. I stepped outside on my back deck to get some fresh air. This small activity tired me out. Recovering from a double mastectomy is tiring. One of my drain sites is bleeding a little but overall my incisions look great. I am seeing Dr. Rock at her office soon. I can't wait to get these drains out. Although I do have some discomfort, I'm not experiencing too much pain, unless the drain tubes get pulled on. I felt honored that a friend of mine presented my name at a breast cancer relay today. I am thankful for all the food, get-well wishes, cards, prayers, and reiki. They help.

May 19, 2019. I stopped taking the pain pills. I was getting constipated, itchy, and drowsy on them. I started using turmeric and ice packs in place of narcotics. I napped quite a bit today; it's like I just had a big thing happen to my body recently. Today was windy and the power went out for a bit. Not the power to heal, though. The healing continues.

Chapter 18

"She wears her scars like a warrior, for they're a reminder she's alive!"—Wallace Stegner

May 20, 2019. The pain has been exceptionally bad today. The thing about pain is that it demands to be felt. I broke down and took a pain pill and laid in bed for most of the day. It feels like my chest is on fire or ripping open. I keep looking under my surgical bra just to make sure that the incisions are not literally opening up, catching fire, or becoming infected. The incisions still look damn near perfect. It must be the nerves waking up. Speaking of nerves waking up, the post-surgery hand numbness was resolved the very next day. Since I cannot move around much, I read the novel *The Fault in Our Stars* by John Green. Spoiler alert—it is about teenagers with cancer who have to navigate just being teenagers, on top of battling cancer. I cannot imagine going through cancer during adolescence. I don't think I even knew anyone personally who went through cancer during the high school years. It's hard enough as an adult. I have come to the conclusion that cancer is very difficult at any age. I have had several patients with cancer in my career. The youngest cancer warrior-patient of mine was twenty-three. I assisted him from pre-diagnosis to survivorship. He had a great attitude through it all. I am realizing that non-physicians make better patients than physicians.

May 21, 2019. I saw Dr. Rock in her office today. Sadly, I could not get my drains pulled out yet. I have a small hematoma (collection of blood) on my left side. The final pathology report came in. They found invasive cancer and micro-metastasis in the lymph node. This means I am going to need chemo. Dr. Rock and I just cried. I am angry, scared, and in total shock. She tells me that this is going to be a tough year. I am especially angry since they said my lymph nodes looked normal on the ultrasound before surgery. They looked normal on the mammogram and on the breast MRI. The fucking sentinel node testing was NORMAL at the time of the mastectomy. My breast surgeon even told this to my husband after she left the operating room. Cancer truly sucks! My case will be presented to the tumor board on Thursday to determine the staging and regimen. My heart is breaking.

As it turns out, the pathology showed not one but three different cancers in the left breast, and it was deemed "unstageable" on the new staging system because of that. On the initial biopsy, it showed Ductal Carcinoma In Situ (DCIS/ stage 0)—breast cancer just confined to the milk duct. On final pathology, I had DCIS along with invasive ductal carcinoma (IDC), which is a type of cancer that ruptures out of the duct, and Paget's disease in the nipple. Paget's disease, named after Sir James Paget, is a rare type of cancer that affects the skin of the nipple and areola. It is a standard of care to check the cancer for hormone sensitivity. My cancer was triple positive: sensitive to estrogen, progesterone, and HER2neu (human epidermal growth factor). Now, I slightly regret taking those birth control pills in my twenties. Maybe this was a risk factor. But I didn't know I was infertile then. Nor did I know I possess a genetic mutation that increases my lifetime risk for cancer.

May 22, 2019. As one can imagine, yesterday was one of the worst days of my life. I decided today that I needed some laughter. I took a pain pill and then watched every episode of *Zack Morris is Trash*, on Facebook. I laughed for hours. I was just following the common advice that laughing is good medicine. Yes, it is heartbreaking and defeating to be told that you have cancer. It is even more heartbreaking and defeating to be told that your lymph nodes look normal on ultrasound, MRI, and sentinel node biopsy, and then get a phone call saying, "Sorry, they [your lymph nodes] are positive for cancer after all. You are going to need chemo." My case was going to the tumor board in two days, a meeting in which my case would be discussed by all the hospital experts. I felt like I had swallowed a boulder. My loved ones tried to be helpful. They told me: "Many women and men have gone through chemo and gotten through it, you certainly can." I was still terrified. They told me, "I think University would take good care of one of their best doctors." I felt like I was going through hell.

Chapter 19

"If you're going through Hell, walk through like you own the fucking place."
—Winston Churchill

May 23, 2019. I am feeling antsy today. Ever since I woke up this morning, I have had the most energy since my double mastectomy. I dusted the top of my dresser. I colored in one of the adult coloring books I had received as a gift. I chatted with a friend. Still, my mind is racing. I keep wondering what the tumor board recommendations were. I will find out tomorrow. It is tempting to log into the EMR (electronic medical record) to see if the tumor board recommendations are in there. I was too afraid to go through with it, though. Oncology, like breast surgery, is outside my scope of practice, and I wanted everything to be explained to me in layman's terms. Tomorrow is the day I should be able to get my drains out. I have an appointment with my breast surgeon followed by an oncology team appointment.

May 24, 2019. The morning started out well. The sun was shining, it was a beautiful day, and it was the morning I got my drains removed. The early morning was only just beginning, though. Marty came with me downtown to the main campus of the hospital for my oncology appointment. The day dragged on like turtles trudging through peanut butter. The oncologist I saw is one of the most respected in the community, and she did spend a lot of time explaining things to me. It was all so overwhelming. I wanted to run and hide. I almost did. But since I had had surgery only nine days ago, running was not an option. I couldn't stop the tears from pricking my eyes and running down my cheeks. I felt like a wreck.

Chemo. The word itself can turn stomachs. Everyone knows that chemo is hard on the patient. I learned a great deal from my team. The team consisted of the oncologist, the oncology nurse, the pharmacist, and a social worker. The standard of care for triple positive breast cancer is a regimen called TCHP (Docetaxol, Carbiplatin, Herceptin, and Perjeta.) This four-drug regimen is given via IV every three weeks for six cycles and gives me the best chance gaining remission. First, I have many appointments between now and the time chemo starts on June 20. I have to go back to the operating room to have a med-port placed for easy IV access. My veins suck and nurses always have a hard time drawing my blood and starting IVs, so the port is absolutely necessary. In addition, I have to have a baseline echocardiogram (ultrasound of my heart). Apparently this regimen can cause cardiomyopathy (damage to the heart muscle) in some patients. I also have to get a CT scan of my chest, abdomen, and pelvis, and a bone scan to see if the cancer has metastasized. Yikes. My head is swirling!

The oncology pharmacist goes over the long list of side effects with me—hair loss, possible nail loss, nausea, fatigue, diarrhea, mouth sores, and loss of taste. In addition, the chemo will likely put me into menopause. In my family medicine practice, I prescribe medication very carefully and conservatively. If a patient of mine has failed lifestyle changes and needs medication for high blood pressure and cholesterol, I tell them to stagger them. I advise them to take one, wait one or two weeks, and then start the other one. This way, if there are side effects, the patient knows where they are coming from. In oncology, it is the opposite. In treating invasive cancer, they give five medications with terrible side effects all at once (in addition to the TCHP, I am prescribed Neulasta to help boost my white blood cells to fight infection). Then the oncology team prescribes four to eight more medications to chase the side effects. There are steroids to prevent drug reactions, multiple nausea medications, and Tylenol or naproxen for pain. Whatever happened to "Do no harm"? It goes out the window in oncology. One of my prescriptions reads, "Total Cranial Prosthesis." In other words, a wig.

Chapter 20

"Keep going, even though it gets harder. The view you seek is beautiful at the top."
—Unknown Author

May 25, 2019. There is not a word in the dictionary that can describe how awful and terrified I feel. I thought I was over my fear since the surgery was supposed to be my only course of treatment. As a physician, I was never taught how to be a patient. I couldn't find a single article on the internet about physicians who have become patients. There is no class on this issue. No medical school lecture. There is a chemo class next week, but this still does not teach a physician how to be a patient. I feel so vulnerable and exposed. Being at the cancer center for four hours yesterday as a patient made me want to jump out of my skin. Seeing these pale, weak, sickly, hairless patients in wheelchairs makes me tremble with fear. All I can think is, OH. MY. GOD. That is going to be me in a month or two. I have to try to keep in mind that I am still in control and that getting chemotherapy is a complete choice. And the side effects will only linger for a short time, not forever.

To everyone who thinks that this choice should be a no-brainer, do me a favor and close your eyes. Picture yourself initially very strong, independent, and financially stable. Picture yourself going from a hard-working, half-marathon running, supermom who rarely misses a beat, to a sickly cancer patient who is now too weak to care for herself or her family. To me, the thought is just horrendous. Again, there is no word for it. In addition to being fearful, I feel sad and angry. As I am healing from my surgery, I am no longer experiencing cancer symptoms. It seems to me it would be much easier to say no to chemo, no to radiation, and no to medications with horrible side effects in this situation. But, without these therapies, I would likely have cancer spread throughout my organs and bones by age forty. This sounds even worse.

May 27, 2019. I cannot state this enough—my purpose in life is and always has been to help others. From age fourteen, when I was volunteering at the hospital, to medical school rotations, I have always showed vulnerable patients compassion. I became a physician to help people. I became the medical director of a family medicine residency clinic to help teach compassion and humanity, in addition to medical sciences, to my medical students and residents. Now I can only hope and pray that my medical team shows me the same amount of compassion and understanding. I realized that, even though I am on medical leave from my career, I can still help others. I read somewhere that everything I am going through can prepare me to be part of someone else's survival guide. I journal and write poetry because I find it therapeutic. A friend reminded me today that I have given so much, but that I also need to receive. I need to let go and give into the universal balance of giving and receiving. It is a deep learning process for me. This is the toughest class yet.

Chapter 21

"And once the storm is over, you won't remember how you made it through, how you managed to survive. You won't even be sure, in fact, that the storm is really over. But one thing is certain—when you come out of the storm, you won't be the same person you were when you went in. That's what the storm is all about."—Haruki Murakami

May 28, 2019. Today I went to see the radiation oncologist. With the exception of the oncology pharmacist, my team is all made up of women. Strong, intelligent, heroic women. The radiation oncologist is recommending twenty-five radiation treatments (five days a week for five weeks) once I have completed chemotherapy. It is less invasive than another surgery to remove lymph nodes. The radiation oncologist has explained that radiation can lower the chance of cancer recurring by thirteen to fifteen percent or so. It is recommended in patients who are young (under fifty), HER2 positive, with positive lymph nodes. My case checks all of those boxes. In addition to valuable information, she also gave me an origami crane stating it was a symbol of healing and hope.

At this point, it seems like this ultramarathon of treatments will never end. Speaking of marathons, I cannot wait to start pounding the pavement again. Dear therapist, I don't need that couch because running is my therapy. When battling through infertility and all during the adoption process, I ran three to five miles every morning before work, and seven to ten -miles on weekends. Two days before Elliot was born, I ran my first half-marathon. That was one of my proudest moments in life. I felt almost as proud that day as the day I graduated from medical school. The race started in downtown Detroit and traversed the Ambassador Bridge into Canada, and then it went back through the Detroit–Windsor tunnel under the Detroit River. Since it has been only two weeks since my surgery, I won't be running tomorrow. However, I will be walking two miles. That's my goal.

May 29, 2019. Today I am going to the wig salon to get fitted for "my rug," as my husband and son call it. I spoke with my brother, Ben, on the phone today. He asked me what the best part of my day was. I told him it was when I cooked vegetarian enchiladas. I couldn't lift the baking dish since I am still on lifting restrictions, but he reminded me that I need to look for the good aspects of each day. Some days prove harder than others. While I heal, I will sure as hell try.

Today was Elliot's last full day of school for the year. Good-bye Pre-K and hello Kindergarten! The memories and emotions of the day we picked him up from the hospital are so fresh in my mind. My hands shook and I could not sit still when I got the decisive phone call on October 22, 2013. I was at work when the social worker from the adoption agency called. I was with a patient but then I saw that I had a voicemail that said, "Youre son has been born. Come to the hospital tomorrow at 1:00 pm with a car seat and a check, and you will get him." Those words are branded on my head and my heart. Being a mom has been one of my greatest challenges, but also one of my greatest joys. Elliot gives my life the purpose and strength to keep going on days when I want to give up. So here I am, moving forward. I am taking it one hour and one day at a time. I have been getting out of the house more, even though I am not driving yet. A friend took me shopping, and I had the makeup person from Saks do my makeup. And I got those damn two miles in that I committed to, although I was walking very slowly.

Chapter 22

"Strength does not come from winning. Your struggles develop your strengths. When you go through hardships and decide not to surrender, that is strength."—Mohandas Ghandi

May 30, 2019. Today was a busy day. I went to school with my husband and Elliot to clean out Elliot's cubby. After that, I had a routine dental checkup and cleaning. By the time the appointment ended, it was time for chemo class. Most of the information presented in the class was very basic like "wash your hands" and "you will probably feel tired." At the end of the class, the nurse gave everyone a tour of the infusion center. I ran into a patient of mine, who was there for chemotherapy, and his mother (also a long time patient of mine). She ran up to hug me and I had to stop her. I cannot be hugged because it will be too physically painful. Then I felt obligated to tell her the truth—that I was just fifteen days post-op from a double mastectomy for breast cancer. I also told her that, in a few weeks, I was going to start chemo there. Initially, I did not want any patients to know about this, but as my journey evolved, I don't mind as much anymore. If my cancer journey can help just one person, it will have served its purpose.

Today I made a huge decision about work. I ultimately decided that it is best if I stay on short-term disability until I complete my six rounds of chemo. I am fortunate to have both short-term and long-term disability insurance. Initially, I felt sort of guilty, but I have to take care of myself before I can take care of anyone else. Chemo affects everyone differently—a seventy-year-old woman can sail through it, while a forty-year-old woman can struggle with serious side effects. I have no idea how it will affect me. There is so much uncertainty, and the uncharted waters are terrifying. I feel like I am about to jump out of an airplane without a parachute. Besides, my OMT (manipulation) appointments are very physically demanding. I would probably miss many days of work due to the side effects of chemotherapy, and I wanted to prevent my patients from having numerous appointment cancellations. I did not make this decision lightly. I weighed out every pro and con and asked friends and family for advice. Like many young "gunner" physicians out there, I never said no. I almost always squeezed patients in when asked. I went into my mastectomy with one hundred and eighty-four unused vacation hours (out of one hundred and ninety per contract year). Now it's time to take care of myself.

May 31, 2019. I am overcome with anger today. I just have to say that, at times, cancer makes me want to punch, hit, throw things, and kick in the fucking wall. However, I am not healed enough to do any of those things yet. Also, it is so damn annoying to me that pink is the color that is supposed to represent breast cancer. Pink is a soft, delicate color. Pink does not represent the grit it takes to have a double mastectomy, go through six rounds of intensive chemotherapy, five weeks of daily radiation, a year of infusions, and then pills for five to ten years. As of today, I am post-op day sixteen. I am healing well. The incisional pain now feels more like a bad sunburn across my chest. I saw my acupuncturist this morning and I will continue to see her weekly. I am so grateful my insurance covers acupuncture. She enlightened me on a type of therapy called "sound bathing," in which you are surrounded by the musical tones of Tibetan bowls. I continue to learn more and more each day.

This afternoon I was visited by an old college friend. She came down from Philadelphia for a long weekend. It was so nice to be outside in the fresh air, and to be able to walk and talk. I am feeling the calm before the storm, or maybe, I am in the eye of the hurricane. Scanxiety (aka anxiety related to cancer scans) is very real and it is starting to creep in. On Wednesday I am scheduled for CT scans of the chest, abdomen and pelvis, as well as bone scans to check for metastatic disease. Since every test I have had so far (mammogram, ultrasound, MRI, and biopsy) has had abnormalities, I could use some good news.

Chapter 23

"The journey of opening the heart wider than our fear takes time and perseverance."—Don Miguel Ruiz

June 1, 2019. I just finished reading one of the most influential books I have ever read entitled *When Breath Becomes Air*. It was written by a thirty-six-year-old neurosurgeon who is diagnosed with terminal lung cancer. He lives twenty-two more months and loses the ability to operate, but he finds what makes his life worth living. There are two parts I keep reading over and over again because they echo my soul. One part states, "As a doctor, you have a sense of what it's like to be sick, but until you've gone through it yourself, you don't really know." How profoundly true this is! I thought I understood what my patients were feeling and going through, but you never truly know until you have experienced a life-threatening illness yourself. The second part that strikes a chord with me is this: "Once again I had traversed the line from doctor to patient, from actor to acted upon, from subject to direct object." Doctor and patient are really two completely different worlds. I believe this is one of the most difficult transitions: to become a patient after you have been a physician. This may have to do with "knowing too much" as someone once said to me, but I think it really has more to do with the contrast between being confident and strong as a physician and the vulnerability and fear you feel as a patient. I am learning this intimately.

Additionally, almost everyone in the world (myself included) says to people with cancer, "You will beat it." Here is some food for thought—that may or may not be true. No one has a crystal ball to tell us if we will live a week, a month, a year, or decades from now. I think that this phrase makes the person suffering with the disease feel like a failure if they end up not beating it. For the record, I am not upset at anyone who has ever said this to me. I, myself, have said it many times. I can remember saying it to my grandfather, who had metastatic pancreatic cancer, a week before he died. This is another conversation that is imprinted in my brain and heart for eternity. When papa said to me, "If I don't make it, my car is yours." My knee-jerk reaction blurted out, "What are you talking about? You're going to make it!"

I am trying my best to navigate things and I feel like I am on the steepest rollercoaster. One moment I am up at the top, the next moment I am down at the bottom. One thing is this, I must continue to learn and transform. I must continue to try to change the world like I have aspired to do since childhood.

June 3, 2019. Today I was able to walk over three miles. The weather was damn near perfect. I had lunch with a friend and then did some walking. I am still restricted to lifting a maximum of five pounds but I have no restrictions on walking. My arm range of motion is getting better. I judge it based on how I can reach up into the cupboard and how well I can dress myself. This three-miles walking has exhausted me and I am heading to bed early tonight. It is hard to remember the days when three miles of running would energize me.

My anxiety is high. It is not just the "scanxiety," I am also anxious about my port placement on June 6. The financial counselor from the hospital called to tell me how much I owed for the tests and surgery. I know she is just doing her job but I just wanted to reach through the phone and scream, "Haven't I been through enough? And now you want me to pay you this much before I can have my surgery?" I did not actually say these things out loud. I just squeaked out an "okay" before hanging up. I understand that many of my emotions are displaced anxiety from this whole journey. I wonder sometimes just how much a human body and soul can take. I read today that a cancer diagnosis is traumatic enough to cause PTSD. I believe it. I will try to not let this journey break my spirit.

Chapter 24

"Death is not the biggest fear we have; our biggest fear is taking the risk to be alive—the risk to be alive and express what we really are."—Don Miguel Ruiz

June 6, 2019. After very little sleep, I awoke at 4:30 a.m. to shower before leaving for the hospital. I had to be there by 6:00 a.m. for my med-port placement. The procedure was minor compared to a double mastectomy. We were back home by 9:30 a.m. I feel foggy from the anesthesia but the weirdest thing is this tickle in my nose. Ever since I got home from the hospital, I've had a constant tickle high up in the left side of my nose, and I cannot stop sneezing. I even texted my surgeon about it. She, too, thought it was strange. I had oxygen delivered via a nasal cannula during the short surgery but nothing high up in my nose. Nasal cannulas are very superficial and would not cause this symptom. What the hell! Shortly after arriving home, I sneezed about one hundred times. I took some allergy medication and used nasal saline rinse, but I still had the feeling of something high up in my nose. I texted a friend of mine who is an allergist (ah! the benefit of having doctor friends!). She recommended a nasal steroid spray and a different allergy medicine. Irritating does not describe the frustration this caused.

June 9, 2019. I was beyond happy when the dreaded nose tickle resolved after a full day. I underestimated the pain I would have from this stupid port. Once the numbing medications wore off, the pain was terrible! At times the pain was far worse than the mastectomy pain. Who knew? I concluded that my body does not like this damn port. I also think that surgeons doing these procedures need to go through them and experience the pain themselves. I realize every person has a different pain tolerance but for me: if the physician states you will have mild pain for one to two days, multiply that number by one hundred to get a more accurate representation.

Some good news is that I had a "normal" test result. I do not have cancer in the bones. I do have some nodules in my left upper lung. That finding wouldn't bother me if it was in the right lung or even the left lower lung, further away from where the cancer was located. My CT scans showed enlargement of the liver and spleen, kidney stones in both kidneys, and a teratoma (tumor with hair, bones and teeth) in my right ovary. My body is weird!

June 10, 2019. Yesterday I was at a birthday party for my son's friend. Another rare, beautiful, perfect day in Cleveland. As I was talking with the other parents, everyone kept telling me, "You're so strong!" Honestly, I don't feel any stronger than anyone else. I am a human, I bleed like everyone else. I have cried like a baby. What exactly defines "strong"? Is it because I put on clothes and makeup and get out in the land of the living for a few hours? Even though there are many times I feel a tendency to pull away from friends and family, today I am out in public. Alone time is good for the health and the soul, with a good balance of togetherness and connection. I don't feel strong at times, when I go from feeling calm to biting mad or when I'm crying. A wise doctor told me today that it's "normal." I hate the word, "normal." There is nothing "normal" about having invasive breast cancer at age thirty-eight. I understand that ups and downs are common to what I am dealing with, but there is nothing "normal" about it. Common colds are common, but not the normal state of health.

Today my oncologist called me about my scans. She consulted with two different gynecology oncologists about my case and this weird ovarian tumor I have. Only one to three percent are malignant, the majority of them are benign. They are scheduling me for an internal pelvic ultrasound. My oncologist was not that concerned about the lung nodules. She sees them all the time. I am already dreading the possibility of having yet another surgery to remove the ovary. Deep breath and focus on the good—no cancer in the bones, high chance of obtaining remission, and loving friends who show up when you need them most. In the words of John Wayne, "Courage is being scared to death, but saddling up anyway."

The Beacon (dedicated to my supportive friends and family)

You are a beacon of light and you don't even know it,
A beacon of hope, and there are so many ways you show it.
Here you stand with a mountain on your back,
Yet you walk forward with a strength that many lack.
If you are tired, you certainly don't show it,
You are a beacon of life and you don't even know it.
That mountain you are carrying, you were only meant to climb.
You are beautiful inside and out, when you smile or when you cry.
Frowning or smiling, you show your feelings so raw.
That is where your strength is, that is what I saw.
You speak your truth so openly and share your fears with the world,
And those who know you, are seeing the shiniest pearl.
You are truly a beacon of hope, love and light.
You don't even know it, but to me it is in plain sight.

Chapter 25

"It's not the amount of days in your life, it's the amount of life in your days."
—Abraham Lincoln

June 11, 2019. The best part of my day was being able to walk fifteen thousand steps today. I may still struggle to get dressed, but I am focusing on what I can do instead of what I can't do. I had my baseline echocardiogram today (heart ultrasound). The tech said it was difficult because of air and fluid in the tissues from surgery. I am still healing. Since I am off work and find myself with extra time on my hands, I do research. Today I found a place that promotes how to heal naturally from cancer. This is right up my integrative medicine alley. Hippocrates Health Institute in West Palm Beach, Florida, is a place where a cancer patient or survivor can go for one to three weeks to detox and recover both physically and emotionally from cancer. For everyone who has said the words, "If I can do anything for you": sure, you can do something, send me here! It is set in a fifty-acre lot and provides a daily buffet of enzyme-rich, organic meals. They have a comprehensive cancer wellness plan that focuses on reducing stress on the mind through nature, breathing, and guided meditation. I imagine they feed you lots of raw, healthy foods, and fresh pressed juices. I have been craving fresh pressed juices since my surgery, especially kale lemonade.

June 13, 2019. Twenty-eight days have passed since my double mastectomy, and seven days since my port placement. I was feeling a tad guilty about walking fifteen thousand steps but not working. Then I went to get undressed at the end of the day and I still needed help. It reminded me why I am still off. I had been thinking of all of the things I can do instead of things I cannot do yet. I can put together some awesome enchiladas but I can't lift the baking dish from the oven. I have concluded I am still a badass warrior who has been getting out of bed and participating in life as much as she can. Cancer may have taken my breasts, but it hasn't taken my legs. Cancer has required me to insert a port for chemo in my body, but it hasn't taken my spirit. Cancer is not a fucking gift by any means, but it did make me realize that there is courage and hope inside of me and nothing can take that away.

June 14, 2019. Last night was the 2019 residency graduation and I got to spend time with all my colleagues and residents. I was so busy socializing that I did not take any pictures. However, there was a photographer there and he took pictures of the entire family medicine group. The hardest thing about working with residents is just when you get to know them and they become as close as family. Then they graduate and leave. I miss them when they go. At the same time, the work is rewarding. They enter residency as interns who lack clinical experience and confidence, but by graduation, they have found their confidence and strong medical knowledge.

I am all for advancing science. I even enrolled in the ReBeCa NIH-funded trial that looks at correlating chemo-related fatigue with cardiac effects and involves cardiac testing. I had my echocardiogram earlier this week and it turned out normal. The CT scan of my chest shows zero calcifications in my arteries. Today was the CPET (cardiopulmonary exercise test). I didn't think I would do that well since I haven't really exercised much over the past month or two, but I did great. I asked the cardiac nurse running the test how long it would take, and he said about seven to twelve minutes. I didn't reach my max heart rate until about sixteen minutes and eleven seconds in—second best of everyone in the study (sixty people)! Woot!

Resting Vitals
BP 110/70
HR 70
Pulse ox 100%
Max HR 176, recovered to 102 within thirty seconds of stopping test. Celebrating victories big and small!

Chapter 26

Sometimes when you're in a dark place, you think you have been buried when actually you have been planted."—Christine Caine

June 17, 2019. Saturday (June 15) was Five Star Sensation, a big fundraiser for University Hospital's Seidman Cancer Center. This event occurs every two years. Over the last ten years, this fundraiser has raised millions of dollars for cancer research and treatment. Under the leadership of Michael Symon, a famous Cleveland chef, this event is always amazing. Marty and I have been to Five Star Sensation four times now in eight years. As I walked in to the fundraiser this year, it felt different; perhaps because I have now held every role within UH—a doctor, a donor, and a cancer patient. This feels serendipitous, just as it did when the breast surgeon who taught me fourteen years ago ended up performing my surgeries. I just have to trust the journey.

Yesterday we drove to Columbus for a mini-trip before chemo starts. I don't know how I will make it through this day. My child went to bed late (10:00 p.m.) and woke up early (before 6:00 a.m.). We came here for the Jim Henson exhibit at COSÍ. This summer we probably won't be able to take a weeklong family vacation like we normally do. Stupid cancer!

Jun 19, 2019. I have a confession. I am not feeling remotely warrior-like this time. Not at all. I am thinking of all the places I could go instead of chemotherapy tomorrow. Just when I thought I had reached a level of acceptance about starting chemo, bam! A horrendous nightmare hits. One moment, I was calm, serene, and participating in life, and then, last night, I woke up sobbing and swearing because of a terrifying nightmare. In this nightmare, I showed up for my first chemo and a bunch of things scared me away from it. And I ran off before they even had a chance to start the IV. I stormed out and never went back. I'm not sure I can do this. Signing the consent form for chemo was one of the hardest parts. It is basically signing an agreement to get poisoned. Poison is defined as a substance that will cause illness or death for the host. Chemo causes major side effects; it is, by definition, a poison. The chemo contract specifically states that my treatment team will respect my decision to stop treatment at any point if I want to. Stop? I don't want to start! There is risk of damage to my heart, liver, and kidneys. Who in their right mind signs this form? Me.

I'm supposed to start tomorrow, but I honestly want to know *why* people show up willingly to get poison infused into their veins.? I have not found a good answer yet. What is motivating about vomiting, mouth sores, hair loss, nerve damage, severe diarrhea, early menopause, and possible organ damage? If anyone has a better reason than "to live", let me know. That one just isn't cutting it right now. I was living just fine until I decided to get that mammogram. Just hear me out! Let me cry it out, scream, and rage on the steroids they gave me, and pray for staying out of the fucking psych hospital!

June 20, 2019. I got through my first chemo! It was a seven-hour ordeal that went surprisingly fast. I felt very sleepy because of the high dose of Benadryl and Tylenol they gave me at first. Then, halfway through the treatment, they gave me the "lower dose" of IV Decadron (steroids), and I had immediate flushing and jitteriness. I could not sit still and I jumped out of the bed and did one hundred squats and sixty lunges. The nurse could not believe it. She had never seen something more ridiculous. If a patient of mine said that they had done this, I would have had a hard time believing it. I tried to warn everyone how sensitive I am to steroids. Try this: listen to the patient; they know their body better than anybody. One of the chemo drugs has a high risk of allergic reaction so in addition to the steroids they pump into you, a nurse sits with you with a toolkit filled with epinephrine and other medications to alleviate a potential allergic reaction. Scary.

Now I am a few hours post-chemo and my stomach is already messed up. Also, I found out I can't get the Neulasta device that sticks to your arm due to my being allergic to latex and sensitive to adhesive. The specialty pharmacy will be delivering it to my house and letting me give my own Neulasta injection tomorrow, so I don't have to make the extra trip back to the cancer center. Yuck! More drugs! I am wondering if this Neulasta is really necessary. It's supposed to raise the white blood cell count to help prevent infections, but all I hear from people about it is that it gives you flu-like symptoms and bad bone pain. This does not sound fun to me. I am honestly thinking of skipping anything I don't really need.

On a positive note—I did it all! I found my warrior spirit and I did it. I cannot wait to see my acupuncturist tomorrow. I am eternally grateful to all my family and friends for the cards, texts, and positive messages. They help *a lot.*

Chapter 27

"Anything is possible if you have enough nerve."—J.K. Rowling

June 22, 2019. I felt okay up until Friday evening. We were even able to go to a movie the day after chemo (*Toy Story 4*). Then, I started feeling tired and nauseous. I woke up on Saturday morning at 4:00 a.m. vomiting. I couldn't keep anything down, not even the anti-nausea pills they prescribed. I ended up in the ER for IV fluids. I feel so wiped out. I can't stand this. How can I go back? I am hoping the worst is over for this round! I am angry with my oncology team for telling me that this chemo regimen "usually does not cause that much nausea," and then I end up in the emergency room puking my guts out. Every person is different with what they can tolerate. My team will be tweaking my anti-nausea drugs for the next round of chemo...that is, if I show up.

June 24, 2019. I tried some natural supplements (CBD oil). I was able to go outside and walk the dog for a short time this morning. The last two days were really rough, so I feel quite accomplished. The esophageal spasms were horrendous yesterday. I'm afraid to eat, but I did okay with a homemade protein shake I made this morning. My stomach is still feeling very sensitive, but I am hoping my stomach will behave tomorrow since I will have visitors over at dinnertime.

Courage. Hope. Strength. Let's get through the day!

June 25, 2019. I took medication and still had diarrhea when we went to the restaurant. I hope no one thought I was bulimic since I had to make about eight trips to the restroom. I noticed there was a woman at the table next to us who was bald from chemo and wearing a headscarf. How come she was not going to the bathroom like I was? When will this end?

June 26, 2019. I had my pelvic ultrasound this morning and I saw my ovarian mass on the screen. The ultrasound technician measured it to be 5 cm, which is a little bigger than the measurement on CT. It is weird. My mind flashes back to the day of my breast biopsy. On ultrasound the tumor was around 2 cm, but on MRI it was 6.6 cm. I am interested to know if more surgery is in the cards. To be honest, I'd rather have surgery than do chemo.

Chemo is the worst! My perception is that other people going through chemo make it look easy. Maybe it's all in my head. This morning I woke up with nausea and bone pain, and not just any minor aches or pains. No one really warns you how bad the Neulasta pain is going to be. My back and hips feel like they are going to break when I get up to walk. IT. HURTS. BAD. You can actually feel your bone marrow expanding and putting pressure on your bones. It feels like your bones are going to explode from the inside out. In a long time, I have not cried as hard as I did this morning. I reported my side effects to the oncology team and they will discuss adjusting or lowering the doses of chemo for the next round. I am grateful and thankful for being off work. There is no way in hell I will be able to work with the nausea, vomiting, diarrhea, and this horrible pain. I can barely walk. I also developed some disgusting skin irritation on my face that looks like rosacea. This is miserable! I just broke down and took some meds to chase these side effects (Tylenol, Zyrtec, Ativan and CBD oil). A nap sounds in order—and soon! I haven't been sleeping well at night either. I figure when all of this is said and done, I am going to New York or Las Vegas and eating my way from one end of the town to the other. I will have earned it.

Chapter 28

"When the dust finally settles, you will be ok. Not like a bright shiny penny, but burnished by your experience. The tests that blur your vision will wash your eyes clean. You will see your worth, more clearly than ever and more precious than you ever imagined."—Margaret B. Moss

July 2, 2019. Being thirty-eight and with cancer is awkward, and let me tell you why—I go to the cancer center and everyone seems much older than me. Everyone my age is in the sandwich generation, busily working, taking care of their kids, and worrying about aging parents. Cancer is not something on the minds of busy working thirty-eight-year-olds with spouses and children. Many people in the cancer center are retirees who have their gray-haired spouse or retiree friends to compare aches and pains with. On the other side of the fence, kids with cancer get tons of sympathy and attention. The kids have their own pediatric centers where the parents can support each other. The kids get to spend time with other kids their age getting treatment. The kids get their wishes granted—celebrity photo ops, commercials for St. Jude, etc. And here I am: stuck in this awkward in-between and with my world flipped upside down. Going from busy working-doctor-mommy to cancer patient at thirty-eight is strange and awkward on so many levels.

My keen level of observation is a gift when I am a doctor, but, as a patient, it is a burden. Nothing will change my emotions. I do appreciate the fact that I have friends and family to support me through this. People I haven't talked to in a while have stepped forward to check in and offer kindness in various ways. I love and appreciate these things so much. I guess there is no normal with cancer and it's probably awkward for anybody going through it. So, I will continue to share my feelings as I move through the ultra-marathon of cancer treatments. Tomorrow and the next day I may feel different. On any given day I feel a variety of emotions.

July 6, 2019. Next week is my next chemo treatment. The thing that makes it so incredibly difficult is that, now that I am seven weeks post-mastectomy and over two weeks since my last chemo, I feel pretty good. I have no symptoms of cancer, but yet I have to walk into a cancer center and get poison poured into my body. The poison is what makes me feel like shit—weak, bone pain, nausea, vomiting, diarrhea, etc. It is the hardest thing to do. And why should I when I feel fine? It is so unfair! I am motivated by all the wonderful men and women who die way too young because of this horrible disease. In fact, I am going to dedicate my next treatment to a lady in my support group. She has stage 4 cancer and she just enrolled in hospice yesterday. She isn't even fifty yet. She has a pre-teen daughter who is facing losing her mom. Cancer is so unfair. It doesn't discriminate. Cancer does not care if you are rich or poor, young or old, or a model citizen. It will bring the strongest person to their knees. And the only thing I can do is take poison. But I will do it next week, for my family and for those who are losing their lives to this horrible disease. I just have to keep going through the good days and the horrible ones.

Today is one of those horrible days. Today I got out of the shower and my hair just started falling out like crazy. I didn't think I would take it this hard. I was told that hair loss usually occurs about two weeks after chemo. Everyone in the world knows that cancer patients often suffer complete hair loss from chemo. What people do not tell you is that you actually feel your hair follicles dying. Your scalp feels sensitive and sore and prickly. It is an awful feeling. I am crying like a baby now. Probably because I was living in denial all week, feeling like a normal human being, and then bam! Reality hits me in the face! This is so hard.

<u>Anger</u>
Screw this awful horrible goddamn disease,
It's only a year they say it will be a breeze.
Stop lying to my face, it's harder than ever
No breasts, no hair, what more can they sever?
Stupid Chemo has now damaged my heart,
I used to be healthy and I want a new start.
I am so hot with anger, I want to scream and yell,
I want the world to know I have been through hell.
Why cancer? Why now? I hate this so much.
I am so hideous my husband won't touch.
No raffle, no dinner, no Go Fund Me page,

It should be easy to see why I am enraged.
I try to calm the fire that burns deep down inside,
Like a volcano, it eventually explodes, but I tried.
It is Roaring, burning, consuming my mind.
When will I be healthy? My spirit I need to find
I want Peace, I want health, I want fucking time,
It's heart-wrenching how life can turn on a dime.
As I fight for the strength to just stand today,
Anger boils, how fucking cancer found a way.
It has turned my world upside down,
And I'm stuck with so much anger now!

Chapter 29

"Even now, as broken as you may feel, you are still so strong. There's something to be said for how you hold yourself together and keep moving, even though you feel like shattering. DON'T STOP. This is your healing. It doesn't have to be pretty or graceful, you just have to keep going."—Maxwell Diawoah

Jul 7, 2019. My hair continues to fall out from the chemo and even though this is expected, it is still devastating, because:

1. Hair is part of your identity.
2. Before hair loss, you look pretty normal and healthy, but after, you definitely look sick (hair loss equates to failing health).
3. It's scary because deep down there is an irrational fear that it won't grow back.
4. It's yet another loss I have to face (after infertility and the loss of both breasts, this adds more to the loss of feeling like a woman).

If you have not realized it by now, cancer sucks. *Please* don't ever tell a cancer patient that "it's just hair." I may have said this years ago to someone with cancer in their past. I am sorry. Only now do I understand how insensitive this phrase was. It feels very dismissive of one's emotions. I honestly didn't know I would take it this hard until it started to happen and I saw handfuls of my own hair in the shower. As I thought about it and analyzed the meaning behind it, I understood why it was so hard. With all these changes to my appearance, I feel so ugly inside and out. I thought that a wig would make me feel better about my appearance. It doesn't. The wig is a cute style and it suits my face, but it is hot and itchy, and it feels unnatural to me. I just want to scream!

Chemo

Loss of taste, loss of hair,
Cancer is truly and utterly unfair.
Stomach pains, throwing up,
Bone pains so deep, can't stand up,
Hot flashes, messed up brain,
Can't recall ever feeling so drained.
Eyes are watery but mouth is dry,
Crazy mood swings make you cry,

Feeling ugly, can't look in the mirror.
A cancer diagnosis causes fear.
Go to surgery to insert a port.
The scar sticks out like an ugly wart.
Watching this poison drip into veins,
Knowing later you will be in pain.
Chemo is not for the mild or weak,
But it is necessary for the cure you seek.
Possible damage to the liver or heart,
You're now a patient with a lengthy chart.
Blood work, X-rays, bone scans too,
It's enough to make anyone blue.
Fighting this disease takes a lot of grit,
Put on the gloves and get ready to hit.
Kill the disease and then gain time,
One day healed, both body and mind.

July 8, 2019. Today I was very productive; I got a lot of things done—I returned a few clothing items, deleted six hundred and fifty emails, wrote some pages in my book, and then went to The Gathering Place for the much needed support. The better I feel, the closer I am getting to the next chemo. I cannot reiterate how frustrating, infuriating, and scary it is to physically feel fine but then to have to walk into a cancer center and have various types of poison poured into your veins. The nine or ten days after chemo are the worst. These are the days when it would be helpful to have things like cards, letters, or even a text message with a corny joke or encouraging words. In addition to journaling, I have been writing poetry as well. Writing has been therapeutic to me.

July 9, 2019. Last night I had terrible insomnia. My soul knew something was amiss, the same gut feeling that indicated to me that something was terribly wrong that night in January 1999 when I raced to the hospital. I did not eat dinner or change out of my *Sesame Street* scrubs from work that evening (I worked in a pediatrics office). That was just hours before my papa took his last breath. In 2005 when I was a third-year medical student, I had the same gut feeling and, because of it, I badgered my attending physician to order a chest CT on my patient who ended up with a dissecting aortic aneurysm. It is the same gut feeling that made me blurt out to my husband "I think I have stage 2 breast cancer" the week before my mammogram. Gut feelings can be guardian angels. But also, it is not a foolproof system. I cannot solely rely on gut feelings as a physician; I, of course, must use my training in science and medicine.

The insomnia and unsettling feeling I had last night may or may not have to do with the death of a fellow physician-mom in my support group... Now I know for sure that I must keep moving forward, no matter how hard it is. Fall down seven times, get up eight.

Chapter 30

"Time is non-refundable, spend it with intention."—Melvin Alexander

July 12, 2019. I am supposed to take steroids the day before and the day of the chemo treatment. Let me tell you about all the ways I hate steroids. The insomnia is the worst; I cannot sleep at all no matter what I do. I am tired but I cannot sleep. And all the worry that goes along with it does not help either. The steroids also turn me into a raging bitch who has no ability to regulate her emotions. Steroids are a lifesaving medication but sometimes they are the devil. In some patients, they can even cause psychosis.

Jul 15, 2019. I feel like I have become anemic because of the chemo. I have felt so terribly weak over the last two days. It's a huge effort to even pick my head up from the pillow. In fact, I am about to head to bed now. It is remarkable how it goes from one extreme to the other—the other night I got no sleep due to the steroids and now I am sleeping so much. Oh well. This is life on chemo. Some days are horrible, some days are just a little bad, and some days are decent.

July 18, 2019. Last night I had the biggest cry yet. I cried for three hours straight. I have concluded that it's not just because of losing my breasts or hair; I am grieving big time. Grieving the loss of womanhood. It is definitive now that I will never carry a baby or breastfeed. I never thought I would say this, but I miss my period. Chemo has put me into a sort of menopause, or "chemopause." I get hot flashes and mood swings. As I have mentioned before, I feel ugly when I look in the mirror. I hate what cancer has done to my body. I hate my flat chest that constantly feels tight. I abhor the chemo and the constant metallic taste, the body aches, the upset stomach and the fatigue. I hate that some people treat me like I am contagious. It is painful hearing and seeing all the maternity photos and baby news. It feels like a slap in the face. The tears flowed for hours. In addition, I feel like I am in this awkward place where I am too sick to work but too well to stay in bed 24/7. Maybe there is something to Mercury being in retrograde, and it's screwing with the natural order of things. I don't know. All I know is that I think I reached my lowest emotional point of this whole journey. It can only go up from here, right?

Today I dragged myself out of the house and I went to a pottery class at The Gathering Place. When I first arrived, I felt like I might burst into tears. And then my mood lifted as my hands worked on the clay. In a way, it reminded me of doing myofascial manipulation on a patient. For an hour and a half I was distracted from my despondent emotions. I even engraved a song lyric on my little pot, "Take these broken wings and learn to fly." Thank you, Sir Paul McCartney, for writing one of the best songs in the history of the universe. I am lucky to have been able to hear him sing these words a few years ago when he toured in Cleveland. As I tell my patients, crying does not mean you are weak. It just means you are a human being with real emotions.

Patience

When a serious diagnosis slows you down,
It is ok to take time to accept and come around.
Be gentle with yourself and take rest when you need,
You must nourish yourself as you plant the seed.
Learn to balance time with others and time alone,
Give yourself grace if you don't pick up the phone,
Punch, kick, scream and cry if you must,
Then pick yourself up and brush off the dust.
It's the little things you find when you slow down,
The little things like finding a coin on the ground.
You have permission to nap if you are tired,
One day your child will look up at you inspired.
Be patient and respect this journey that you're on,
Even when think you are weak, really you're strong.
Live without fear even if the prognosis is poor,
Take time to recharge, renew and restore.
Beauty surrounds you if you take time to notice it,
The softness of your pillow or a candle that's lit.
If nothing else, learn patience to get through each day,
Patience and gratitude will help pave the way.

Chapter 31

"It's ok to cry when there's too much on your mind. The clouds rain, too, when they get heavy."—Amina Mehmood

July 20, 2019. I am slowly adjusting to my appearance. I am completely bald now. Just when I was feeling I had reached my emotional rock bottom of this whole journey so far, I bounced back. Only the universe knows why. I feel that there were many factors, not just one thing. Crying and venting was probably therapeutic. Yesterday I got acupuncture, spoke with my counselor, and then went swimming for a little while. I have to wear a long-sleeved rash guard, long swim leggings, and a hat to protect my sensitive skin from the sun.

Today I got dressed, I put on makeup, and I got out of the house and saw some friends. In addition to my family and friends, I have also been in contact with other women physicians with cancer in my private support group. They help lift me up. Many of them are in chemo right now and they are also bald. It is interesting to me that some women feel bold-and-badass bald. I am borrowing some of their courage (I may not give it back!). Some women feel sad-and-insecure bald. I am more of the latter. I never leave the house without a hat, turban, or wig.

July 22, 2019. Other than the unrelenting hot flashes and loss of taste, I am feeling quite well today. I had lunch with a good friend who has experienced her own share of losses. Then, I went for a walk by the lake today because I was early for an appointment to have a post-mastectomy lymphatic massage. Even though it was just Lake Erie and not the ocean, being by the water helped my mood. After my time in nature and my massage, I feel as amazing as one can feel under these circumstances. I am viewing my baldness differently now. I see it as a gift given to me to help counter the hot flashes. My husband pointed out the similarities between this and the scene in the movie, *Napoleon Dynamite*, where his friend, Pedro, gets hot and shaves his hair off. I couldn't help but laugh. Feeling satisfied and thankful for this good day.

July 24, 2019. Has anyone ever noticed before that all the emojis on smartphones are bald? How come I never noticed this before? Now I can finally make peace with my baldness. Today, Allergan, the company that makes breast implants and tissue expanders announced a big recall of their products. I have never been more relieved to be "flat and fabulous." Thank you, gut feelings, for helping me avoid these implants.

July 26, 2019. This morning I met a doctor from my support group for brunch. We have so much in common. We are both thirty-eight and have children at the same school. She trained as a neuroradiologist, but she hasn't worked since being diagnosed with stage 4 lung cancer in 2017 (her prognosis at diagnosis was six to twelve months). It's a beautiful thing that she was able to get into a clinical trial that has halted her disease progression, and she is still alive to this day. I envy that she has been able to let go of the natural physician guilt of not working; I have not. It's hard for me to find purpose outside of identifying as a physician. But we both agreed that the hours and stress of working are bad for the disease. Part-time physicians work forty hours a week; full-time physicians more like one hundred. Anyone who is a physician, married to a physician, or has a family member or friend who is a physician, knows that the work is intense with high burnout rates. In fact, just before being diagnosed with cancer, I had been working on an abstract on physician burnout and the high rates of suicide in the profession. I had also attended Robyn Symon's documentary, *Do No Harm*, at the Cleveland Film Festival this spring. When I am reminded of this, I am able to let go of some of the guilt. It is now time to care for myself. Nobody ever gets to the end of their life and says, "I regret not working more."

Once I am done with the "big chemo" (intense four-drug regimen, five if you include the Neulasta shot, which has horrible side effects), I still have the "little chemo" (IV Herceptin and Perjeta) every three weeks for a year *and* twenty-five sessions of radiation; then, estrogen blocking pills for five or more years (or a lifetime). The research and guidelines change every few years, so it is hard to know what the future recommendations will be. I know one thing: I will never be the same person after this. Hopefully, I will be someone who puts herself higher on the priority list than she used to; and I will conceivably use those PTO hours for vacations and not surgeries or chemo. A part of me does worry that I will go back to being overworked.

Chapter 32

"Without my struggle, I would have never stumbled upon my strength."—Alexandra Elle

July 27, 2019. I am taking advantage of every good day. This weekend I went to dinner and to a play with my husband. Unfortunately my stomach was on the fritz, and I had to walk out of the play about eight times to go to the bathroom. Stupid chemo! I ended up standing in the back of the theater with the ushers to minimize disturbance to the other theatergoers. Tomorrow I will have another lymphatic massage, see my oncology team, and have blood work. Then, in two days, I will have three out of six procedures from the "big chemo." The oncology NP told me that the regimen I am on is one of the most difficult chemo regimenss.

July 30, 2019. On an interesting turn of events—the negative pressure hood at the pharmacy in the satellite location I get chemo at is broken, and I have to go to a different location for chemo. I'm happy that my chemo nurse, Jen, is being sent to the other satellite office, and she is going to do my chemo. Silver linings.

July 31, 2019. I am now halfway done with chemo. I didn't take any steroids this time and I feel so wiped out already. I had acupuncture before chemo this morning to help with the hot flashes and nausea. Also, a friend stopped by and sat with me for a while. With our busy schedules and lives we had lost touch over the last year. There are some friends with whom you can go years without talking, and then you can pick up right where you left off.

Today's Stats
Height: 5'5".
Weight: a number between 100 and 200.
Hemoglobin: 10.6 (normal 12-16) anemic.

August 2, 2019.
I wanted to write a poem today,
The words escape my chemo brain.
Sleeping a lot, feeling so weak,
Must keep going and reach the peak.
I can, I will, I tell my mind,
That warrior spirit I will find.

August 4, 2019. In the last three or four days I could barely eat anything because the nausea was so bad. And, even when the nausea isn't bad, I cannot taste anything anyway. I can taste sour foods like sour candies and lemonade, and that's about all. It is quite sad. In my physician-cancer support group, one of the ladies had a dream about having long, dark hair (she is also bald due to chemo). However, in *my* dreams, I dream about food. In one dream, I couldn't wait to dive into a soft-serve hot fudge sundae and taste it. In another dream, I have a massive gyro sandwich. In real life, I have an overactive sense of smell and I cannot stand my favorite frankincense soap right now. But at the same time, I have no taste or a constant metallic taste in my mouth. Chemo does weird things to you.

August 7, 2019. Over the last few days, water tastes like an ashtray and I can only taste sour foods like lemonade and sour candies. Although, weirdly, carrots and hummus tasted good to me yesterday. Maybe it is because there is lemon juice in hummus? I appreciate the thoughtfulness and the offers I have gotten for home-cooked food and my favorite treats, but it just frustrates me so much that I won't be able to taste it or enjoy it. I will take a rain check. I will be researching the best restaurants in the country. I want recommendations for when my taste and appetite do come back. Until then, a girl can dream.

August 9, 2019. Eight days after chemo is usually my turning point for feeling better. I have to admit, round three kicked my ass. Literally and figuratively. I had a little bit of energy this morning and took a nice walk. It felt so good to get out in this perfect seventy-degree weather. My life feels Sisyphean. It's as if I reach the top of the mountain, carrying a giant rock, and then I get pushed right back to the bottom.

August 11, 2019. I read this very accurate article today entitled "Angels and Bolters." When I was first diagnosed with cancer, someone told me that the people you thought you could count on may abandon you. And then people you barely know will come out of nowhere to help you. I have found this to be pretty accurate. Cancer does not just change you; it changes your friends and family members too. To sum up this article, loved ones can be categorized as a Preacher, a Clueless person, a Bolter, an Angel, or a Fellow Traveler. Preachers are the ones who give you advice.

Said advice could be about anything—a diet, a supplement, how to pray, etc. The ones who are clueless are the ones who have foolish things to say: a remark about why you got cancer or about cancer being a gift. Give me a fucking break. The bolters are the people you thought were your friends, but who disappeared when you got cancer. They always have an excuse like they were busy or they thought you needed rest. Angels are the ones who are always there for you to pick up things at the store, or drive you to an appointment, or offer to watch your kid. Fellow travelers are those who want to be there for you, but don't know how exactly.

My skin has been horrible over the last few days; my eyebrows are sparse and it takes a lot of effort (more makeup than I usually wear, and my wig) to look decent. As I mourn the loss of my breasts, my hair, my beautiful skin, and my thick eyebrows, I cherish my time with my family and walking my dog. At least Pooh Bear doesn't seem to care about the drastic change in my appearance. The moral is—there are always things to be grateful for (angels and fellow travelers, you know who you are).

Warrior
Hey Wonder Woman, can you lend me some strength?
Cancer has me down and the smile is hard to fake.
I call myself a warrior, a goddess, and strong.
But deep down I am sad, this journey is long!
I have wanted to quit so many times down deep,
I want to be honest, the hill is so very steep.
I was terrified of surgery and sad to lose my breasts.
Now that part is over but still I cannot rest.
Since I started chemo I have lost more than my hair—
My heart function has declined and given me a scare.
I have thrown up more times than I ever have before.
Been in the hospital for blood transfusions and more.
I have missed out on time with family and friends.
Sometimes if feels as if this battle will never end.
But I pull myself up by my bootstraps each day,
Wishing and hoping that in the end, I'll be okay.
So I will Warrior on and take it hour by hour,
Never mind, Wonder Woman, I have found my lost power.

Chapter 33

"I think it's brave you get up in the morning even though your soul is weary and your bones ache for a rest. I think it's brave you keep on living even though you don't know how to anymore. I think it's brave that you push away the waves rolling in every day and you decide to fight. I know there are days you feel like giving up, but I think it is brave you never do."—Lana Rafaela

August 13, 2019. I have been missing work somewhat. I miss the patients I was used to seeing regularly. Work, as hard as it is sometimes, gives me a sense of accomplishment and purpose. For the first time in a month, I logged in to my email. I productively went through all six hundred eighteen emails. And then I signed up to give a lecture in February. In order to help myself get back in work mode (still eight weeks away), my therapist recommended I read some medical literature. And behold: I find this depressing article that points out that chemo damages your DNA and bone marrow and makes you more likely to get leukemia in the future. Highest-risk cancers were bone and testis; breast cancer was lower but still with an increased risk. Colon cancer did not infer an increased risk.

To get through this, I imagine Elliot in his Tae Kwan Do sparring gear, as the chemo and my body literally kick the cancer's ass. Watching him at martial arts is entertaining. It makes me want to go back to kickboxing. Maybe one day...

Chemo in 8 days!

August 17, 2019. Yesterday was a good day. We walked around the Akron Zoo for a couple of hours. I was exhausted by the end of it and I could barely move. My oncologist encourages walking, even when it's hard, to offset the bad effects of chemo on the body. Elliot wore his *Ghostbusters* costume and captured some ghosts at the zoo. He got a lot of compliments for his attire. I wish I had his courage to be bold and not care what people think. I am dreading my next chemo on Wednesday.

Here's to burning cancer to the ground!

Rise Up

When a bone breaks, it grows back stronger.
Hang in there, Gabby, just a little bit longer.
Healing and good times are just around the bend,
Even though you can't tell yet, you're on the mend.
You will soon be back in the gym burning away the stress,
Feeling the sweat drip down as you run your very best.
The insomnia and uncertainty you feel will be overcome.
When you get what you long for, life is rewarding and fun.
So stop any pity party, you are better than that,
Rise up to the challenges and step up to bat.
You have so much to offer, so many gifts to give,
The bumps in the road you are facing will be short lived.
Don't let fear stand in your way,
And always give your best each day.
When you get knocked down, you must get back up.
When you are feeling empty, just take time to fill your cup.
You are so strong, you have proven that so many times.
You can do anything you dream if you continue to try!

August 20, 2019. This morning I was happy to be in my third week of chemo cycle, on the day before my next chemo. This is when I feel my best. I have to share the excitement and experience of dropping off a kindergartener for the first time. Elliot is comfortable at his school, and I think this year will be good for him. He has half days all week, and then, next week, he will start his normal 8:30 a.m. to 3:00 p.m. schedule. This afternoon I went to acupuncture and had my blood work drawn. Now I am waiting to see my oncologist at 2:40 p.m. I'm dreading tomorrow. Chemo seems so much harder than my surgery was; so many ups and downs and weird side effects. On some days I get a rash, crazy eyelid twitching, watery eyes, or a constant runny nose. Why don't they tell you about this in chemo class? If I can be thoughtful and reflective for a moment—even though I miss my patients, I am glad I took this time off work. I would feel guiltier to have my staff cancel patients left and right because I am too weak to get through even a reduced schedule.

August 22, 2019. Yesterday was chemo number four out of six sessions. I am weak, partly from being anemic and partly from the chemo itself. I think recovery from my surgery was easier in some ways because each day I am improving little by little. Chemo wipes you out and then, by the time you are almost at your healthy baseline, *bam*, you're knocked right back down again. It is dreadful and it is so hard to go through. I am planning to go to the infusion clinic tomorrow for some IV fluids to see if this helps the nausea and weakness. Just two more of the big chemo treatments and I'm done. Then I get twenty-five radiation treatments and the "little chemo" for a year. Just have to keep on keeping on!

Chapter 34

"Courage is not having the strength to go on; it is going on when you don't have the strength."
—Theodore Roosevelt

August 23, 2019. Yesterday afternoon I was hit with a strong pain that felt like a Mack truck smashing into my right kidney. I have never had a kidney stone in my life but the pain was agonizing. My husband called EMS to transport me to the hospital where I was admitted with a 6 mm obstructing kidney stone, and with swelling in my right kidney causing intractable nausea and pain. I'm also dehydrated and too nauseous to drink or eat, so I'm getting plenty of IV fluids. Now I am waiting on the urology department to see me. How much can one person take?

August 24, 2019. Still admitted. I am having surgery around 12:30 p.m. to break up the kidney stone with laser lithotripsy, and to possibly place a stent in the ureter to hold it open. Still getting waves of terrible pain and nausea. I am miserable! Worst. Year. Ever.

August 25, 2019. I am recovering after yesterday's emergency surgery to open the blockage from the kidney stone. It was a bad blockage, and my right kidney was swelling and starting to shut down. Now I will have a stent in my right ureter until Tuesday. It feels like I am sitting on razor blades. Riding home from the hospital in the car was awful. My blood work wasn't good this morning and the internist wanted me to stay until tomorrow morning but we compromised and I stayed until 5:30 p.m., long enough to eat and get some more IV fluids with added magnesium, potassium, and calcium. I didn't eat for three days, you would think I'd be starving but I am not. I'm glad to be home in my own bed with my own shower. Having this stent inside of me has made me completely incontinent, with malodorous, blood-tinged urine, and I am wearing a diaper. This kidney stone thing has to be the most painful, but also the most humiliating thing I have ever been through. I am still weak and anemic (hemoglobin 7.7; the normal numbers should be between 12 and 16), partly from chemo, but I may have lost some blood with the surgery. Here's some advice—do not get an obstructing kidney stone ever, but especially not when it's the day after chemo! This whole situation was torturous. I can't wait to get this stent out of me. Tuesday can't come soon enough (stent removal day). Hoping to stay out of hospitals for a while. Here's to getting stronger and better each day!

One thing I cannot understand is why none of my doctors sent me home with a prescription for pain medication. They told me to take ibuprofen. You have got to be kidding me. I know we are in the middle of an opiate epidemic, but I am a cancer patient who just had surgery for a kidney stone—the worst pain there is next to labor contractions. Now, I am not a fan of taking a lot of medications, but there is a time and a place for prescribing pain relievers. While prescribing opiates has fallen dramatically over the last few years, more people are dying of opiate overdoses than ever before. I wonder if not treating pain appropriately leads people to run to the streets for heroin. It crossed my mind.

August 27, 2019. I had my stent removed today. The urologist said I could remove it myself, but I was not comfortable with that. He also said that I would be in pain for a few more days because of the trauma to the kidney, ureter, and bladder. I am getting bad pain in the area of my right kidney that comes and goes. He did an X-ray today which shows that the stone is gone. I just wish the agonizing pain would be completely gone too. I was discharged from the hospital without any prescription for pain medication, and over the counter medications have not helped much over the past couple of days. This pain was far worse than anything I've ever gone through in my life, worse than any broken bones or surgeries. I have concluded that chemo plus kidney stone equals disaster.

August 29, 2019. My bone marrow is not really working, my blood count has dropped even lower now (hemoglobin 7.1) and I am feeling very weak. My oncologist had me come to the cancer hospital today and get IV fluids and a blood transfusion. Initially, I felt horrified to watch two pints of O+ blood drip into my veins. Blood outside of your body is nauseating to see. To me this is scary, but everyone here keeps telling me it will help me feel better. Honestly, I would like to stay out of the hospital. This has been the shittiest week ever, and, to make matters worse, I'm too sick to attend my brother's wedding in Florida. I am heartbroken. I feel like the most useless bridesmaid in the world. I have missed the bridal shower since it was a few days after my chemo treatment. I have missed the bachelorette party and, now, I have missed the wedding. This is devastating me, I cannot remember ever being so sick in my whole entire life!

August 31, 2019. Yesterday was a bad day. I was sick with vomiting and diarrhea, and I am still passing kidney-stone fragments. I guess this can go on for weeks after lithotripsy. I honestly feel so bad for anyone who has ever had a kidney stone.

I heard this quote recently and found it very appropriate: *"And this too shall pass. This rough patch may pass like a fucking kidney stone but it will pass! Thinking positively doesn't mean you won't go through tough times it means you know that there will be good days ahead."—Author unknown*

September 2, 2019. I had some very brief periods of nausea and pain today, but I've been feeling much better than over the last ten days. I was even able to take a little walk and do some light cleaning today. My cheeks are pink again. Between the blood transfusion and my bone marrow working again, I am feeling physically better. (Just in time for chemo to knock me on my ass again next week.) Summer of 2019 is coming to an end soon. It was a shitty summer but I did get to the pool a couple of times in my sun hat, long-sleeved rash guard, and long swim leggings (chemo makes you more sensitive to the sun).

September 4, 2019. I have less than a week to go now until my next chemo. I am feeling tired today so I took an afternoon nap. I'm not lightheaded like I was when I was very anemic. I wonder if my bone marrow is holding up okay. I will have my blood drawn on Tuesday to check everything. I need my platelets to be above 100 and my hemoglobin to be above 8 to go ahead with chemo. If I am out of range, I could have an extra week off... we will see. Tomorrow is parent night at Elliot's school. It will be my first outing in weeks (other than to hospitals, doctors' appointments, and the pharmacy)! I am feeling a little self-conscious about it since I now have no eyebrows or lashes left. Losing eyelashes is annoying by the way. They go into your eyes! This is the shit no one warns you about. They really need to add this to the curriculum of chemo classes. I cannot wait until this is all just a distant memory.

Chapter 35

"It's ok if you lose your spark. Just as long as you rise as the whole damn fire."
—Colette Werden

September 6, 2019. I am fighting through fatigue, hot flashes, insomnia, and irritability today. The nonstop fun of cancer treatment and early chemopause never seems to end. I hate that I am exhausted but cannot sleep. I am thirsty and water tastes like piss at times. I have no strength and my brain is like mush. Don't get me wrong, I do have some good moments when I can get outside for fresh air, a walk, lunch with friends, a good quality nap... Let me be reminded of good times when I'm going through such intense bad times. Must. Keep. Going.

September 9, 2019. I have been so physically tired over the last couple days. This is weird because normally I have an increase in my energy in the days leading up to chemo. I have been able to walk the dog in the mornings, which is good. I think the hot flashes that interrupt my sleep may be a factor. I am listening to my body and relaxing now, watching a movie.

September 10, 2019. I am feeling like the American poet and political activist, Alice Walker today who stated, "People tell me I am strong but I am so, so tired!" My day has been filled with appointments today—acupuncture, oncology team appointment, labs. My oncologist says my body needs more time to recover from the rough patch involving the kidney stone and the blood transfusion. So tomorrow I will only get the two monoclonal antibodies (Herceptin and Pertuzamab) and not the chemo meds (Docetaxol and Carbiplatin). I may be done with those chemo meds entirely since there is no research study that proves six is better than four rounds of TCHP. I haven't decided yet. Right now I am so medically traumatized from everything. I need more time to recover and process all of this. If I do decide I am done with the "TC" part of it, I only have sixteen more "little chemos" left!

Drowning

With oncology appointments, scans, treatments and more,
Like waves that wash over me...but where is the shore?

There are so many things that go through my head each day,
the feelings of oppression, I wonder how long they will stay?

Drowning in helplessness when I can't get out of bed,
Feeling some days like drowning in water over my head.

Drowning with anxiety that feels like a weight on my chest,
Each and every day I give more than my best.

If you care to listen, hear me now when I am raw with emotion,
I am overwhelmed, fighting a current out there in an ocean.

Every morning I wake up, I never know how I will feel;
will the waters be calm? The uncertainty is real.

One day I'm in the hospital getting a blood transfusion,
I'm lightheaded and dizzy and feeling confusion.

One day I wake up in the morning feeling strong and fit
But then I get a call from the nurse and the bad news hits.

My heart is weak from the treatments to fight cancer;
Will I be able to get more chemo? I don't know the answer.

The cancer I have is an aggressive kind;
I am only thirty-eight, I am not ready to die.

I tend to bury my anxiety and have kept this fear of death inside,
But I am swimming against the current now with nowhere to hide.

Some days I am drowning—my fears are an ocean so vast;
Some days it is hard to stay afloat and the water swells fast.

I swim toward the shore, swim for my life feeling like I will drown,
But I have made it through today although tears may trickle down.

I look forward to the day when I make it breathless to the shore,
For now I am alright and I will continue to do my best and more.

Though the water is deep and I feel as if I am freezing,
What is waiting on the shore is warm and it is freeing.

I did not drown ånd have made it through another day.
Sometimes the shore is nearby and other times far away.

Today is a gift. When I stop struggling I float.
Sometimes I am alone, sometimes with a full boat.

As the waves move up and down, I may smile or shed tears,
But today I have not drowned from the cancer or my fears.

September 11, 2019. I couldn't have gotten the hard-core chemo drugs today even if I wanted to. I found out my platelets were too low: 94k (normal 150-400); they have to be above 100 for the Docetaxol and Carboplatin. My blood count is also still pretty low—hemoglobin is 9.3 (normal 12-16). Still, 9.3 is better than 7.1, which is what I had the day they gave me a transfusion of two units of blood at the cancer center. Several people suggested I take iron. I'm not bleeding and my iron level is actually high, so it would not be helpful to take iron; it may actually cause more harm than good. So they only gave me the monoclonal antibodies today. It was a short chemo day. I shouldn't feel as horrible as I usually do with the Docetaxol and Carboplatin on top of the Herceptin and Perjeta. Also, I don't need the Neulasta shot when I am only on the H&P. This makes me happy since the injection makes me feel like my bones are breaking, and my body feels like lead. So, for now, we will reevaluate at my next oncology appointment on October 1.

September 13, 2019. It is lucky Friday, the 13th! After four months of applying and waiting, I have finally been matched with Cleaning for a Reason. I got a phone call this morning that I am entitled to four hours of free cleaning services for having cancer. It's my prize for putting up with this shit show all summer. It's my lucky day, and it's Friday the 13th, and a full moon today. It would have been more useful to have this service when I was recovering from my bilateral mastectomy but beggars can't be choosers. Everyone in the medical field and in the teaching field—hang in there! I have received many cards in the mail and I am feeling immense gratitude for all the positive thoughts, vibes, juju, prayers, love, messages, and cards. They are helping me get through this rough patch (the roughest patch) in my life.

September 14, 2019. I spoke too soon about having good luck on Friday the 13th. A bad storm hit our little city and we lost power at about 8:30 p.m. last night. The sky was like something out of *The Wizard of Oz*, so Elliot and I slept in the basement. The power is still out. Huge oak trees are uprooted; grocery stores and gas stations are closed. It's almost like a tornado hit our city but they are calling it a "microburst." Our little suburb of Cleveland even made the national news and weather channel. We are going on almost twenty-four hours without power now. The happy news is that there were no reported injuries or deaths. Cars and roofs can be replaced, but people cannot. My gratitude is high today. My energy is still a bit low, but I cannot complain. It's a beautiful day today!

"I'm not saying I'm Wonder Woman, but nobody has ever seen me and Wonder Woman in the same room together!"—Author unknown

September 16, 2019. Life is one big, giant, crazy adventure, isn't it? After the powerful Friday storm we have been without power ever since (this is day four). I read Elliot stories by flashlight last night. Luckily the weather has been perfect—not too hot, nor too cold in the house. I feel like my energy is improving and I am hoping my bone marrow is finally recovering. When it rains it pours! Literally and figuratively! I had to throw out all of the food in the fridge and freezer. Ironically, right after I did that, a colleague who lives a few streets over from me offered up his fridge and freezer to put our food in. Oh well, our fridge got a nice deep cleaning for the first time since we moved here in 2008.

September 17, 2019. The power is back on. I wish I could use said power to jump-start my brain. I am suffering from chemo brain really bad. I wonder if the bit of stress with the power being out made my chemo brain worse; I had already been having difficulty with word finding and naming actors, for example. Then, this week, I almost ran a red light while driving, I couldn't find a restaurant five minutes away from my house to which I had been before, and I missed an appointment this morning. The chemo brain has been bothering me. I wonder when this will go away, but hopefully it will be soon! I need my brain.

September 20, 2019. I am agonizing over a tough decision: should I try to get in two more rounds of TCHP (aka "big chemo")? As you recall, I had to skip round five due to low blood counts. Or do I stop at four? According to my oncologist, there is no published research stating six cycles are superior to four, but then why does everyone else get six cycles? Oncology is so foreign to me. This would delay my return to work by about three weeks, but it is not a huge issue as I have disability payments coming in. What to do? I am feeling torn.

"Wisdom is nothing more than healed pain." —General Robert E. Lee

September 22, 2019. My son (a month shy of turning six) just came up to me this morning, put this cape on me and said, "You can be the Hot Flash and your super power is shooting hot flashes from your hands!" If anyone can make hot flashes funny, it's Elliot! Now to chill and watch the Detroit Lions blow it in the football game. And here's the cancer update for the weekend: I am about ninety percent decided about going back to full chemo to get the full six rounds. This way, no matter what happens, I can have the peace of mind knowing that I did everything I could to stay on earth. Invasive HER2 positive breast cancer (the kind I was diagnosed with) is much more aggressive than HER2 negative and the ten year survival rate is about fifty percent. This is nothing to mess around with.

September 23, 2019. I just got a call with bad news that my echocardiogram showed a significant drop in my EF (ejection fraction), and I have to now see someone from cardiology on Thursday and possibly modify my therapy. The ejection fraction refers to how much blood the ventricle of the heart pumps out in one beat. The normal amount is fifty-five to seventy percent; mine is now about forty-five percent. Apparently, this happens for a small percentage of women who take Herceptin, which is why they do a pre-chemo echo, and then follow up with echocardiograms. I will potentially have to start taking heart meds, but I will know more Thursday. This is bullshit. Screw cancer!

September 24, 2019. I have just had my annual eye exam and I am happy to report that my eyes have gotten a smidge better since last year. So I finally have some good news to report after all the crappy news. It is ironic that the moment I make the big decision to go for the full six chemo cycles, my heart decides to get weak, and, as a result, I might get taken off chemo anyways. But I have good eyes! It's all the better because I am able to see the beauty around me.

Chapter 36

"She wears strength and darkness equally well, the girl has always been half goodness half hell"
—Nikita Gill

September 25, 2019. October is now just a few days away and stores will be awash with both pink for breast-cancer-awareness month, and orange for Halloween. Please be mindful of all the "pink washing!"

1. The famous Susan G. Komen foundation raises millions of dollars and is one the best-known charity organizations. But did you know that only twenty percent of the money raised by the foundation goes to breast cancer research?

In comparison, eighty-eight percent of the money donated to the Breast Cancer Research Foundation actually goes to breast cancer research.

You can check out these sites before donating to see how charities are rated: Charity Watch or Charity Navigator.

2. Please think before you Pink! Check out: www.thinkbeforeyoupink.org for tips. Here are some things to know:

   - Many companies have already decided on the amount of money they will donate to the cause, no matter how many items of a particular product are sold.

   - Don't buy things that have the pink ribbon if the product itself is known to cause cancer (i.e. KFC, certain perfumes, etc.)!

   - Avoid items with the breast cancer ribbon if they will not specify how much of the proceeds go to the cause and which organization. There are so many!

3. You're better off giving to a respectable charity rather than wasting money on a product you don't really need. Or just give me the money! (I'm joking, of course.)

September 26, 2019. I saw the cardio-oncology nurse practitioner today.

I guess they have a protocol for patients that develop heart issues on chemo.

1. They will do echocardiograms more frequently (monthly).

2. I can continue Herceptin and I have to take a heart medication—a beta-blocker called Carvedilol, which I should be able to drop whene I am done with the treatments.

3. If I become symptomatic with congestive heart failure (CHF), or if my ejection fraction drops below forty percent, they may have to hold the Herceptin or come up with an alternative medication

YUCK—more meds. F--k!

By the way, the number one cause of death in cancer survivors is not cancer. It's actually heart disease.

September 29, 2019.

"Hot flash" (a short poem)
It's not a hot flash, it's a power surge.
Bring on the water, here comes the thirst!
Menopause at thirty-eight from chemo is unfair.
The hot flashes are worse than the loss of hair.

September 30, 2019. *"Talking about our problems is our greatest addiction. We should talk about our greatest joys." —Rita Schiano*

I'm remembering last September when I went to a leadership conference for women physicians at the Cleveland Clinic. One of the main themes was building each other up. I was listening to Dr. Sasha Shillcutt, founder of Brave Enough (BE) and author of the book, *Between Grit and Grace: The Art of Being Feminine and Formidable*. Sasha started the organization to empower other women physicians in their careers. Women who were fighting to balance in their careers and in their lives. She was correct in saying women physicians work their asses off and often seem to be in competition over who had it worse. This is true in my own life. When I see my colleagues at a work meeting, conference, or dinner program we are always talking about how hard we worked, how awful call was, how we saw a million patients, etc. If someone were to say, "I got ten hours of sleep last night, had a wonderful morning with my family, and an easy day at the office," we would be mad as hell at them (out of pure jealousy). Well, I have had a couple of good days and I am going to talk about it.

Sunday evening my husband and I had an amazing dinner date. I had vegan Caesar salad and a vegan pasta dish with carrot bolongnese. Today, after Elliot's eye appointment, Elliot and I had a little squirt-gun fight in the backyard. We then lay down on our towels to dry and look at the clouds. We saw a seahorse, monsters, and a volcano in the cloud shapes. I am so thankful for these moments! If Olivia Newton John, Shannon Doherty (and over one hundred fifty thousand other women in the U.S. living with metastatic breast cancer) can find joy or purpose in their days with stage 4 breast cancer in their bones, then I certainly can do so too.

Tomorrow I will see my oncology team and have chemo. Finding joy will be much harder in the next few days. It's time for me to push that boulder up the hill (again).

On Joy

Some days I feel none,
Some days I have some,
On rare days I am overcome,
With joy.

There are days I have no pain,
When the sun beats out the rain,
When I have so much to gain,
There is joy.

The simple things of the day,
Like a great meal on the way,
Spending time with my family,
That is joy.

Trees lose their leaves in the fall,
But they still stand proud and tall,
There is a season for us all,
For joy.

Battling through cancer now,
Wanting to know why and how,
The treatments have got me down,
Where is the joy?

Some days I can stand,
Or offer a helping hand,
One day walking through the sand,
Smiling with joy.

"It takes courage to say yes to rest and play in a culture where exhaustion is seen as a status symbol."
—Brene Brown

October 2, 2019. I didn't get chemo yesterday because of a scheduling error. Going in for the big chemo tomorrow instead. All four drugs. I'm inspired to carpet bomb the shit out of this cancer after educating myself on HER2 positive breast cancer, which is more aggressive than HER2 negative. A surprisingly high percentage of patients diagnosed early will be re-diagnosed later with metastatic breast cancer (MBC). Jaw-dropping. My blood count was pretty decent, although still slightly anemic (hemoglobin 10.4, normal 12-16). I took my first dose of heart medicine last night and slept like a baby. I wonder if it's going to be like this every night (only time will tell).

Some exciting things happened yesterday! I found out Rothy's shoe company is giving free pairs of shoes to breast cancer patients and survivors. A friend of mine nominated me and I am getting a free pair of $145 shoes made from recycled water bottles. I am also on the waiting list for Magic Hour, a company that gives free photo sessions for cancer patients. Every day I learn something. Cancer School is in full swing!

October 3, 2019. I did my makeup and drew in eyebrows to look pretty at chemo today. Today is treatment five out of six TCHP. I am wearing black because I don't see the color pink as having any grit or toughness. Black is as tough as nail color. It's October 3, three days into "Pinktober" and I am already slightly annoyed with certain advertisements that blame the victim, charities that pay their CEO a higher percentage than the cause, and the sad reality that over two hundred thousand women in the U.S. are diagnosed with this horrible disease. Cancer is not my fault but there are so many articles out there that tell you if you eat right, don't smoke, don't drink or do drugs that you will prevent the disease. I call bullshit! If that was the case, my father who smoked for over forty years, drank soda every day and ate bacon would have the disease and not me. End rant. Here comes my infusion nurse. Let's do this!

October 4, 2019. Today I am wiped out because of the chemo, so I will be making a permanent indent on my couch. It gives me time to reflect and write. As I was getting my chemo yesterday, I heard a couple of patients ring the bell, which meant they were finished with their treatment. The bell is a bittersweet thing. It represents heartache for those metastatic-cancer lifers who will never ring it. But it also symbolizes hope and new beginnings for those who have completed treatment and are NED (No Evidence of Disease). I am still debating if I will ring the bell? And when? When I finish the "big chemo" (TCHP)? Or do I ring it when I finish next year's treatment with the "little chemo"? There are also twenty-five radiation sessions somewhere in the middle. Do I ring it with each accomplishment?

The dilemma of ringing the bell reminds me of being in the hospital when a baby is born and the entire hospital paging system plays a lullaby. It is a symbol of joy for the family who has just had a healthy baby born, but a painful reminder to the patients who have suffered the loss of a baby. Since I will need to take pills for years to prevent the cancer from returning, I feel a little bit like a fraud ringing the bell. That is, if and when I decide to do it. To ring or not to ring, that is the question...

Chapter 37

"Give. But don't allow yourself to be used. Love but don't let your heart be abused. Trust. But don't be naive. Listen. But don't lose your own voice." —Unknown Author

October 6, 2019. I have been hanging in there since chemo. Still feeling pretty weak and tired. Having some waves of nausea that come and go. I would rate this round of chemo as probably the best one yet (knock on wood).

Tomorrow I see the gynecology-oncologist in the morning to talk about my ovaries, or as I like to call them, *useless*. To BSO or not to BSO, that is the question of the day (BSO means bilateral salpingo-opherectomy, a surgery to remove both tubes and ovaries). Then, tomorrow afternoon, I get my cardiac MRI. So far I am tolerating the little old lady dose of heart medicine they have me on. As we go into the first full week of Pinktober, I hope you will do one thing for me: check your breasts! Men get breast cancer too! In fact, Beyoncé's dad was just diagnosed recently with breast cancer, so the PSA is for everyone. Vegan health nuts get cancer too.

October 7, 2019. I ran around UH main campus today. The gynecology-oncologist wants to remove my right ovary, which has a benign-looking mass on it, along with both Fallopian tubes. She would leave my left ovary for my health. The plan would be to shut down my ovaries with medications and put me into menopause for five years. At age forty-three they would take away the medications and let my ovaries start to work again. They may but they may not. It is a crapshoot. By suppressing my ovaries for five years, the risk of cancer recurrence is reduced, especially since my cancer was sensitive to estrogen. Recent research shows many ovarian cancers start in the tubes; so, only removing the tubes lowers the risk for ovarian cancer. The cancer lessons continue. I also had my cardiac MRI today and I won't know the results of this test for several days. While I had some time today, I was reading an online medical journal, and I came across an article from a friend I met online who also struggles with a serious medical condition. She published a short article that made me want to shout "YES!" out loud. It is about learning to give up control and learn how to ask for help from your friends. Ceding control is never easy. It seems impossible to me to let friends help in the way the article recommends. All my friends are busy with work and families. We are all in the sandwich generation with husbands, children, aging parents, and jobs. Trying to manage it all is not easy. But then again, the world does have seven billion people. If that doesn't tell you we weren't supposed to do it all alone, I don't know what does!

I will always keep moving forward. In the words of Dr. Martin Luther King Jr., "If you can't fly, run. If you can't run, walk. If you can't walk, crawl. But, by all means, keep moving."

October 9, 2019. I practiced good self-care yesterday. I indulged in a facial and got some vitamin injections (D, B6/B12). I hope they help my skin issues. It must have been fate that I couldn't log in to my work computer to see the results of my cardiac MRI. I am looking forward to seeing my family this weekend. Come hell or high water, I will be in Detroit, Michigan for my brother's local dwedding reception. I am still saddened because we did not go on any vacations this year. I pine for the day I can travel, eat without abandon, and just have a good time without worrying about sickness. I visited a friend with breast cancer today. It's nice to connect with another person, especially when that person is also a physician with breast cancer.

October 11, 2019. My free Rothy's shoes came yesterday and they fit perfectly. It's another one of those silver linings in all of this mess, one of those little things that can cheer you up on the bad days. And the company has saved over thirty-five million plastic water bottles from ending up in landfills. Who knew? We will be driving to Detroit this afternoon right after Elliot gets out of school. Send positive juju that I will be ok on this trip!

October 13, 2019. I had a great time with my family this weekend celebrating the newlyweds. I hadn't seen my brother in over a year. I dressed to the nines, and mingled with family and friends. I also danced a little and pretended to be normal. I have a great ambition in life: to die of exhaustion rather than boredom. My legs feel so weak today and I am pooped. If you ask me today if it was worth it, my answer will be a strong and resounding "YES!" I even gave a speech for the one hundred and thirty people who attended. My brother's wedding was almost as dramatic as mine. The bride and groom had to move the wedding up a full day because of Hurricane Dorian. The hurricane was expected to make landfall on the evening of September 1, 2019. The only people flying from Detroit to West Palm Beach that Friday were the people attending Ben and Betsy's wedding. And one news anchor! He made sure this made the news on television and in print with the headline, "Couple Scrambles to get Married Ahead of Hurricane!" Never a dull moment in our lives! The funny thing is that the hurricane ended up slowing down, destroying the Bahamas, and never even hitting Florida.

In other news, coming up this week, I have another echo on Tuesday. Tune in later this week for the results.

October 14, 2019. My legs still feel like Jell-O and I am very tired after the trip to Detroit. And my stomach was having a bad day today. My body just needs rest. Still no regrets! I still can't believe my little brother is married and that I have a sister-in-law.

I found out today that *Elephants and Tea*, a magazine for cancer patients and survivors, is going to publish one of the poems I submitted to them. First a poem, and, one day, I will publish my book. Elliot has already come up with a great title. A family friend of ours, Kathy, will be getting one of the first signed copies and a mention in my Pulitzer Prize speech for believing in me.

October 16, 2019. (*Note: a version of this was published by KevinMD and The DO journal online*).

I have to get something off my chest (no pun intended, I've had a double mastectomy). In the midst of "Pinktober," I am bombarded by victim-blaming articles and posters. They all imply that breast cancer is preventable by a healthy lifestyle. "Don't smoke, don't snack in the middle of the night, don't eat sugar, don't eat fast foods, don't breathe fumes, don't live in a polluted area, exercise, don't be overweight, eat broccoli, use turmeric, drink moderately, stay calm, stay positive, get mammograms, drink tea, make sure you get vitamin D, don't use a dry cleaner, eat salmon, etc."

How many cancer patients could fill up an entire page with all the things we've been told would have, could have, even should have prevented our hearing those awful words, "it's cancer"? I know I could.

Here are some facts for you: I did not eat fast food. I didn't smoke, drink, or use drugs. I ran, walked, and did yoga. I drank green or herbal tea every morning. I didn't drink soda. I was the one eating my veggies and drinking water or tea. I ate almost completely vegan for nine years. I am not saying I was perfect, I wasn't. I ate candy and I was a little overweight. Really, my only vice in life was chocolate, but I have read articles stating chocolate is supposed to be anti-cancer. I tried to avoid chemicals whenever possible. I didn't dye my hair and rarely wore nail polish. We even use an organic, food-based, kid- and pet-safe fertilizer on our grass. I was only thirty-seven when I was diagnosed and not even due for my first mammogram (USPTF guidelines say fifty but ACOG recommends forty). I wasn't perfect, but no one is! I used birth control pills in my twenties. Maybe that had something to do with it? I will never know…

It turns out you can have every risk factor and never get cancer. And you can have zero risk factors and get cancer. It's very random. You can have a normal mammogram that misses signs of cancer on the imaging. STOP. BLAMING. VICTIMS!

There is a myth, which claims that, if your cancer is caught early, it will be curable. There are several different types of breast cancer. Some types are more aggressive than others. Some breast cancers are driven by estrogen or progesterone hormones, and some are not. Someone can have more than one type of breast cancer at once. I had three different types of breast cancer found in my left breast—DCIS (Ductal Carcinoma In Situ/cancer confined to the duct), Invasive Ductal Carcinoma (cancer that ruptured out of the duct), and Paget's in the nipple. I got checked out just days after symptoms developed and I find myself with a ten-year survival rate of fifty percent.

Cancer does not discriminate. It doesn't care if you are ultra-rich or ultra-poor. Cancer strikes the ultra-religious, atheists, and everyone in between. Babies get cancer and so do the elderly. Vegetarians and meat eaters get cancer. Physicians get cancer. Let me say this again—cancer does not discriminate. It's an awful hand to be dealt for anyone. So please, let's stop blaming the cancer patients for their diagnosis, and support them in any way we can.

"The truth will set you free, but first it will piss you off." —Gloria Steinem

Chapter 38

"You'd be surprised who is being inspired by your journey. Don't quit!"—Noelle Mae Lumb

October 17, 2019. I am pining for a happy medium. Hello friends and family and thanks for tuning into another week of *what else can go wrong!* Let me explain... After I got back from Detroit, I came down with a cold and sty in my right eye. Of course being on chemo has wiped out my immune system, so it progressed to asthmatic bronchitis and cellulitis of the eyelid. I swear this shit can only happen to me!

I am also waiting on a plan of care for my heart. Had my fourth echo on Tuesday and the results weren't great. As a physician and a patient, I logged into my computer to check my results. They are disappointing.

I have had four echoes (heart ultrasounds) so far. These are my ejection fractions:

1. Echo 1 (Pre-chemo Baseline)/ June 2019: normal 60-65%
2. Echo 2 (July): 55-60%
3. Echo 3 (September): 45-50%
Started Carvedilol (beta-blocker/heart medication).
4. Echo 4 (October): 40-45%

Sadly, the EF just keeps dropping. The ejection fraction (EF) refers to the amount, or percentage, of blood that is pumped (or ejected) out of the ventricles with each heartbeat. Fifty-five to seventy percent is normal.

I am supposed to stay on Herceptin for a year (until June 2020) but if my EF drops to forty or below I will have to take a break for a while or stop it completely. I was told that this was one of the most important medications to treat my cancer and it is scary to think of stopping it. I will wait to hear from my team, but I am guessing they may want to increase the beta-blocker dose or start a second heart medication.

Here I am, laying it all on the table—I am going to vent for a minute! Warning: swear words ahead.

Why the fuck do I have to deal with all this? This journey has been like my life—it's a complete rollercoaster ride! It is the biggest ups and downs followed by upside down loops. It is full of moments that drop your stomach and take your breath away. It's Sisyphean, as I mentioned before. In Greek mythology, Sisyphus was the king of Ephyra. He was punished for his deceitfulness by being forced to roll an immense boulder up a hill, only for it to roll down when it nears the top. He was destined to repeat this action for eternity. So here I am: one minute I am dancing and having fun at a wedding reception, and then, a few days later, I am in the urgent care for bronchitis and eyelid cellulitis.

I have experienced several traumatizing moments in my life. I was in a bad car accident just before my seventeenth birthday. I was driving home from work, stopped at a light, and a drunk driver rammed my car at high speed. It is amazing I came out of that only with minor injuries that have healed. I am not a cat but I wonder some days: how many times can I escape near-death experiences before I actually pass on? That was a good life lesson. I have never driven my car drunk before or after that and I never will.

I don't know what is worse sometimes—physical or emotional trauma. Emotionally, I felt the worst heartache I had ever experienced six years ago when we adopted a baby and then he was taken away from us on day eight. One day I was experiencing extreme joy, and the next day extreme pain. It feels steeper than a rollercoaster—skydiving maybe? I can't just catch a common cold; I have to get three different types of breast cancer at once. Let's just have a happy medium for once for fucks' sake!

"To that soul reading this, I know you're tired, you're fed up, you're so close to breaking but there is strength within you even when you feel weak. Keep fighting."—Author unknown

Getting Back Behind the Wheel

The hardest thing to do once you have been near death
Is to get back up and take in a deep breath.
When a drunk driver hits you and you're only sixteen,
You're terrified, you're injured, waiting for help on the scene.

Scared beyond scared, being strapped down to a board,
You're alone, it's dark, and blood pressure drops to the floor.
Being in shock without your mom or dad there,
Ambulance flying down to the hospital for care.
The nurses in the emergency room try to help you through.
The pain is intense and the fear of death is brand new,
A feeling you have never felt before.
You have no idea what the future has in store.
By the stroke of great luck, the injuries will heal,
But the toll it takes emotionally is the worst part of the deal.

Sitting in court with the drunk driver on the stand,
All you can visualize is the badly totaled van.
You freeze like a deer does when caught in the headlights,
Feeling like you are in that shock again, just like that night.
Getting back in the car again behind the steering wheel,
Heart pounding, wondering if this is how you will always feel.
After a while driving is not so scary or bad,
You're back in the routine that you have always had.
Then a few years later driving home for college break,
You are driving along a high bridge across a lake,
Traveling the left lane driving next to the wall,
Your tire blows and the car spins out of control
The airbags deploy and as the car flies around,
The hood flies up, you pray that you will not drown.
Another lucky day, you are fine, just really scared,
Feeling sad that you've totaled another car in your care.
Should you worry about your driving or feel lucky to be alive?
Emotions swirling with so many conflicting feelings inside.

And then it hits you: you've been in this place as a child.
A driver who ran a red light, driving wild...
Your brother was four and you only eight.
Your mom and your brother were injured that day.
Rushed to the hospital by ambulance that day,
You were not hurt but your brother has two broken legs.
You teach him to walk again and remember that well.

Thirty years later it is so hard for you to tell
With what you have inside of your brain,
Even at times when you know you are safe,
Internally you have fear that leaks into place.
As you care for your patients who are feeling afraid
(They may have even suffered a car accident that day),
You feel a connection with all their fears and worry.
They can tell when you listen with care and don't hurry.
A tragic thing to have had to go through all these things;
Strange how your memories are as clear as a bell rings.

So many thoughts and feelings in your head,
Usually you ignore them and keep busy instead.
With other tough things in your life you've been through,
Car accidents aren't the only memories in view.
Getting back behind the wheel can be really hard,
Or showing up to work the day after you break your arm,
Or returning to work right after you have just lost a baby.
Everything that occurs big or small drives you crazy.
Be brave, warrior, in the ugly face of fear,
Keep moving forward as long as you're here.
Chin up, princess; don't let that crown slip,
And get back behind the wheel in life, that's a tip.
Even when your heart is beating out of your chest,
Show up for life, girl, it is all for the best.
When your motivation falls low, it can only go up.
Get back behind that wheel without fear, but love,
Take care of yourself and know it's ok to cry,
And get back behind the wheel; it is worth it to try!

Trust me.

October 18, 2019. Some thoughts on bravery:
Friends and family keep telling me that I'm very brave and strong.
Everyone keeps saying that I will get through all this. I wish I had a
crystal ball to tell me so. And a magic wand, while we're at it, to make
it all go away, because deep down inside I feel like a fraud. It's true—I

feel fake often. I know it makes people uncomfortable to know the truth, so stop reading now if you're one of those people. Let me lay it all on the table for you. Under my wig (or hat), I am currently bald. Under my clothes, I am wearing an ugly mastectomy bra with silicone prosthetic boobs that make me sweat like a freaking pig. These things were advertised to wick heat away from my body. I call bullshit! Under that bra is a flat chest with two long horizontal scars where my natural breasts used to be. I have to draw on my eyebrows each day to look "normal." I could die from this. It makes most people feel better to say, "You'll be fine! You're a fighter! You are so strong! You're a warrior!" Maybe I will be fine, but maybe I won't. When it comes to cancer, I have concluded that almost everyone says the wrong thing at times. Me included. I am not angry about that—I would rather have my friends say those things than nothing at all. I know they mean well and that it comes from a loving place. When people you are used to talking to on a regular basis just stop talking to you because of a medical condition, that is a very isolating place to be. No one on Earth knows my timeline. I am fighting advanced breast cancer. This cancer kills forty thousand women per year. However, I will continue to be brave for myself and my loved ones. I will be brave as I let my doctors operate on me to remove my breasts and ovaries, pour poison into my veins, burn my skin with radiation, and put me into a chemical menopause. I will take pills lifelong that will weaken my bones and affect my brain. I will do whatever it takes because that's what you do when you're faced with the big C. In addition, I will continue to put on a smile and dance and appear to be in good spirits despite the pain and the suffering. Why? Partly because I am afraid the truth will drive away my loved ones when I need their support and love the most. It is strange for the patient to have to comfort the people around them, but it's what we have to do. More cancer lessons. People need to be reassured that you are okay. Besides, that's what I have a support group for. I can vent and cry with these women when I need to. I can tell them the truth. I have wanted to quit so many times. I almost did. More than once. I didn't want to do any of this—the surgeries, the chemo, the radiation. But I do it hoping to avoid an early and painful death. Is this what bravery is? Suffering in silence because the truth hurts? Is bravery putting on fake boobs, fake brows, and a wig so I'm not an eyesore?

The dictionary definition of bravery is "the quality or state of having or showing mental or moral strength to face danger, fear, or difficulty; the quality or state of being brave; courage showing bravery under fire." Mental strength? Is it mental strength that, even though I took time off work, I don't sit in a corner, curled up in a ball, sobbing my eyes out? I rest when I need to, but I try to take walks and follow the doctor's recommendations. I'm not a horrible patient all the time!

I will continue to face danger—sometimes with a smile and sometimes crying, kicking and screaming—because I am brave.

Finding Strength

She didn't have to wake up, she'd been up all night.
Steroid induced insomnia, up at 3 a.m. with no end in sight.
She is lying there with this deep desire,
A desire for sleep, for she is so very tired.
She is the same person, although with no hair,
Same wife and mommy-doctor with gifts to share.
As she fights to cure the cancer deep inside,
She feels scared with a deep fear she could die.
Her friends and family tell her that she is brave and strong,
But scary thoughts haunt her and say, "they may be wrong."
She doesn't feel brave when she is too weak to stand.
For the first time in her life she needs a helping hand.
She is so used to being independent and stable,
Now it feels cancer has robbed her of all she is able.
It has robbed her of her breasts and of her hair.
Some days the heartache is more than she can bear.
But she still shows up each day despite the pain.
There are some days where the sun beats out the rain.
Any woman who has the ability to walk through this,
To go through surgery, chemo, and radiation has pure grit.
Tomorrow the sun will still rise and still she will be here,
Although she looks quite different when she looks in the mirror.
Deep down she is still amazing, courageous and strong,
And she will find that strength and prove it like she has done all along.

October 21, 2019. Let's talk about all the war terms used when it comes to cancer. We hear it constantly in conversation, in articles, in obituaries. I see it on t-shirt logos, magazine covers, and on TV. I, myself, have been known to use such phrases. How many times have you read something that goes like this: "Jane (or John) Doe has lost their battle to cancer?"

When a cancer patient begins their treatment for cancer, the war language starts. "Gabrielle is fighting cancer" or, "She is battling cancer," or, "She is going to kick cancer's ass!" This language permeates articles, conversations, and obituaries everywhere. When a cancer patient reaches remission, they are told that they have "won the battle." So, does that make individuals who never achieve remission or those who die from cancer losers? I would like to argue that it's not about winning or losing a battle or a war, but rather that cancer is a disease process. It's an unpredictable, messy, scary, and horrible disease process. But that is what cancer is—a disease. My friends and family members who have died from this disease are anything but losers in this made-up war. They were parents, spouses, friends, and wonderful human beings. Wonderful humans like my grandfather, Papa, who passed away from pancreatic cancer in his early sixties. Like me, he was way more into loving and helping others than fighting. He underwent chemotherapy and radiation to treat his cancer. The pain he tried to hide from his face while undergoing treatment was hard for me to watch as a seventeen-year-old teenager. Cancer patients come from all sorts of different backgrounds. Some cancer patients are just babies. I'd like to argue that babies and war terminology do not belong together in the same sentence. Some cancer patients are gentle, peaceful, and loving, while others may be sarcastic and tough. Cancer is not a war, a battle, or a fight. When you're in the thick or it, it is painful and tiring and scary. Maybe that is why so many liken it to war. Cancer is a disease process that happens to have death as an unfortunate consequence sometimes. I just wonder sometimes when, where, and how all of this war language started. I don't hear these battlefield terms nearly as often when someone has heart disease or succumbs to a bad infection. I am not innocent here. I have also used war language many times in the last six months with my own breast cancer treatments. It is ingrained in all of us. It's written in the fabric of our culture. I can't say this strongly enough—soldiers in war are so highly respected and commended, even if they do not make it home. I don't get that feeling with cancer. Those who have succumbed to the disease are just as honorable, than the survivors. The first step towards change is acknowledging what we are doing and saying. Before cancer, I would have not have thought about the fact that battlefield terms are not appropriate. So whether I live or die from cancer, please know that I have lived, I have loved, and I have also learned. I have undergone all the necessary tests and treatments for the disease and the complications that go with it. Just know this—I am not a winner or a loser in this fabricated war.

October 22, 2019. Wish me luck at the doctor's appointment today. My husband seems to think I should be admitted since I have been tired and my heart rate has been high. I actually feel better today than I did on Saturday when we went to the theater and my heart rate was 125 when I sat down, after walking just a short distance. I don't recall having these heart symptoms before with prior rounds of chemo. I am seeing the doctor in about an hour. Stay tuned to see if I can get chemo tomorrow or not.

In my spare time, I have been researching scholarly articles about cancer. I have found over eight hundred and ninety-six articles on a recent PubMed search of Berberine and Cancer. Berberine is an herb that has been used since 2000 B.C. Why am I only hearing about this now? Metformin, an old diabetes drug, is also helpful in cancer treatment apparently according to four thousand and six hundred PubMed articles. I am intrigued since these medications cause a lot less side effects than chemo!

Maybe I will do integrative oncology in the future. It's just a thought. There must be a purpose to this journey, right?

October 22, 2019. Sadly, I have to skip chemo tomorrow due to low blood counts.

White blood cells: 4.8K (normal 4-10)
Hemoglobin: 8.1 (normal 12-16)
Platelets: 62K (normal 150-450)

The plan is to recheck my labs and possible chemo in a week. Chemo is supposed to kill the cancer, not the host. But a wise friend of mine has told me that if it is making me feel this unwell, just think about what it is doing to the cancer cells. I am, however, annoyed with all these complications. I am going to acupuncture now to try to stimulate my bone marrow. One woman in my support group told me to try jumping jacks to stimulate my bone marrow. I can only do three without feeling like I am going to die. Fuck.

October 24, 2019. My heart rate has been high even after taking the prescription beta-blockers, which are supposed to lower it. My cardio-oncologist ordered a fourteen-day Zio Patch to monitor my heart for the next two weeks. Luckily, I can shower with it on! You could only wear the older Holter monitors for up to forty-eight hours and it was a big clunky box with a bunch of wires coming out. The new Zio Patch is just that—a patch. As I mentioned previously, my heart function has fallen to forty to forty-five percent on echo (the normal rate is fifty-five to seventy percent). Between this and being very anemic, I just think my heart is beating faster to try to oxygenate my cells. My dad had a cardiac catherization the same day and has communicated to me that he doesn't need a "zipper job," just a stent. I wonder if my heart beats harder because of the stress. I worry about returning to work. I worry about my mom who needs a lung transplant. I worry about my dad who has heart disease. I worry about my child and my husband and the stress I am putting them through. I worry about my friends and family members who have dealt with their own serious health issues and trauma. I worry about my own heart that is stressed and stunned from the chemo. I worry about my bone marrow and the risk of leukemia developing. I worry about my future. Will I live a long life or will I die young? Tell someone not to worry and that is a sure way to increase their worry. I will have happy moments, despite my worries, and I will try to find a balance of doing what I can to heal. So here is to just living one hour and one day at a time—with or without worry. I hear that stress is bad for you anyway.

October 25, 2019. Today Marty and I celebrate our eleventh wedding anniversary. If you include all the years we dated, we have been together for nineteen years. We will always remember October 25, 2008. A few months before that date, we were planning to travel to Las Vegas for a medical conference. We decided to kill two birds with one stone and get married at the same time. It was a week filled with firsts. It was Marty's first plane ride. Neither of us had been to Las Vegas before. I know what you are thinking, but we did not elope. We had fourteen loved ones attend our wedding.

Marty and I flew in to Las Vegas in the morning, went to get our marriage license, and then checked into the Palazzo Hotel. He stayed behind to nap in the room while I made my way down to the Flamingo Hotel where our wedding was to take place. I had my dress, nylons, shoes, and makeup packed into a small rolling suitcase. I started making my way down the strip toward the Flamingo. Just before I got to the Flamingo, I was pushing my way through a crowded block party at Margaritaville. That is when somebody shot me with a BB gun on the Vegas strip just hours before the wedding. Although I had to make a police report and get checked out by the paramedics, the wedding went on as planned. We have lived and loved each other through a lot during our time together.

I take the fact that my chemo was cancelled this week to be a blessing in disguise. Tomorrow I will be able to enjoy a nice anniversary dinner at Lola's downtown instead of suffering with post chemo side effects.

I am still trying to find a balance between doing too little and too much. Yesterday, I went to an indoor trick or treat at a nearby mall with Elliot and Marty, and today I was so worn out I spent a lot of time on the couch and napping.

Here is the plan for the week.

Monday: Acupuncture (trying to stimulate my bone marrow and treat my hot flashes).
Tuesday: Blood work and my counseling appointment.
Wednesday: Blood transfusion if my blood counts are still low. If counts are good, last chemo!
Thursday: Happy Halloween!
Friday: Alternate chemo date.

Chapter 39

"I smile because I have survived everything the world has thrown at me. I smile because when I was knocked down, I got back up."—Unknown Author

October 27, 2019. On Gratitude:

It can be hard to practice gratitude, especially when you're suffering. Here I am though trying to do it.
I am grateful for:

- My wonderful health insurance. I've racked up probably a million bucks in medical expenses but my out-of-pocket has been under $5000.

- Having access to excellent medical care. My heart breaks for my fellow sisters-in-cancer who have to travel a considerable distance for treatment, or those uninsured patients who don't have access to treatment until it's too late.

- My physician-mom cancer-support-group ladies who know what it's like to go through this and have their world flipped upside down, their roles shifting from doctor to patient.

- My long-term disability insurance I bought when I was still a medical student in my twenties. I am now collecting on this to help pay the bills and I don't have to exhaust my savings, go into debt, or declare bankruptcy. I heard on NPR that forty-two percent of cancer patients cannot afford their medical bills. It's heartbreaking to me to read this statistic. Here you are, sick as hell, and then you get punished twice as hard with extreme financial stress. The undue stress on top of cancer is not a recipe for healing. This will not change until we have medical care as a right, and not as a business built to bloat the pockets of the CEOs of insurance companies. Listen to me: you must buy the best medical insurance and long-term disability insurance you can afford. If you have cancer, there are even cancer policies you can purchase BEFORE you get the disease. They are totally worth the investment. Do it now, especially if you're young and healthy (when the premiums are the lowest). Even if you are a healthy, plant-eating, exercise freak you can get a life-changing disease.

Cancer is a classroom and I continue to learn as the student of a class I never wanted to enroll in.

October 28, 2019. Not every cancer center has a bell. For example, Memorial Sloan Kettering in New York, one of the nations most well-known and well-respected cancer centers, does not employ one. Not only is it heartbreaking for those with metastatic disease whose treatments will never end, it could also be psychologically damaging to those who will recover and survive their cancer. This article, "Researchers uncover dangers of ringing a bell to celebrate 'victory' over cancer," by Eric Lindberg explains why. Cancer cells can be microscopic, lingering dormant in the body stunned by the treatments but still there. Even though the patient has No Evidence of Disease (NED), it could resurface. The future is never promised. Ringing the bell may never be the end.

It's like Pavlov's dog, but instead of salivating at the sound of a bell, some patients solidify the PTSD flashback response to it. It makes sense to me scientifically.

October 28, 2019. What makes a woman a woman?

Is a woman still a woman without hair, breasts, and ovaries? In the words of Erin Brockovich, portrayed by Julia Roberts in the movie, says, "Yes, you are still a woman. A happier woman who doesn't have to worry about maxipads and underwires." But I wonder, is it the way she carries herself? Is it the way she nurtures her family? Is it the way she walks? Is it the way she talks? Is it the way she sees the world? Every woman is different. Some women wear dresses and heels, while other women wear pants and loafers. Some women rock out to heavy metal and others prefer classical music. Some women wear their hair long and others prefer shorter styles. Some women are nurses, others are engineers. Some women are the breadwinners of their families and others are stay-at-home parents. Some women are leaders, others are dreamers. Some women are athletic, whereas others are content to cheer them on from the stands. Women are not just their body parts. Women are special. Despite all their differences, there are traits that all women have in common. One thing is that they are better physicians. No, really! Research indicates patient outcomes are slightly better when the physician is female. Perhaps it is because women are gifted with deeper empathy. There is no doubt women are unique beings. They are not defined by their breasts, or lack thereof.

Save the women! Not the boobs, tatas, or any other vulgar word for breasts. Women can live without them and, if they have cancer, the breasts have to go. Sorry not sorry. End rant for the end of Pinktober.

This being said, I am still in shock that I have gone through the amputation of both breasts. Without the gut instinct that led me to my diagnosis, I would most likely be dead two years from now.

October 29, 2019. It feels like the calm before the storm. Over the past couple of days, I have been feeling better. On Monday I got a methylated B6/B12 shot which boosts my energy so much. And I think this has also helped prevent chemo-associated neuropathy. Today I felt well enough to attend yoga for cancer patients at The Gathering Place. The yoga there is extremely gentle, it can be modified to be performed in a chair, and even people on oxygen participate. It is nothing like the hot vinyasa yoga I used to do at my gym, where the room was heated up to ninety-two degrees, the flow was intense, and people were casually doing handstands.

In addition, I've been seeing an acupuncturist whose niche is oncology. She used acupuncture to help stimulate my bone marrow and it worked. I will able to avoid a blood transfusion tomorrow. My hemoglobin came up from 8.1 to 8.7 and my platelets have come up from 62K to 138K. I can tell because I am not getting so lightheaded or short of breath anymore. My heart rate has been close to my baseline, and I don't feel as fatigued as I did before. I will be getting my last TCHP ("big chemo") tomorrow. Then I have a conference with Elliot's teachers. I was supposed to be a week post-chemo by now. This will be interesting since they usually give me Ativan as one of my three anti-nausea pre-chemo medications before they give me the actual chemo (believe it or not, it helps with chemo-associated nausea). Of course it makes me groggy. I am holding onto hope.

Chapter 40

"Now every time I witness a strong person, I want to know: what darkness did you conquer in your story? Mountains do not rise without earthquakes."—Katherine MacKennett

November 1, 2019. I have been feeling pretty horrible over the last few days. I had chemo the day before Halloween. Chemo is scarier than Halloween will ever be since you never know how bad you might feel. I missed Elliot's Halloween parade at school. He went as Ironman this year—a last minute decision for him. Marty took him out trick or treating, and he had fun in the wind and drizzle. And in true Cleveland spirit, it started to snow overnight; perfect timing for satellite radio to kick off the Christmas music. (Yes, they did). Today I still felt super weak and lightheaded and nauseous, so I went to the cancer clinic and got some IV fluids. It helped a little. I'm now stuck with an icky bitter metallic taste in my mouth. I tried the old home remedy of eating some of my kid's Halloween candy (sour patch kids). Unfortunately the relief was short lived. I'm hoping tomorrow will be better.

November 3, 2019. Round six, my last round of chemo, has been rough on me. Friday I went to the outpatient cancer clinic at Seidman for IV fluids. This morning I woke up with a pounding heart, and I became lightheaded and short of breath while walking through the house. Of course the on call doctor told me to go to the ER (I would have told my patient calling me with these complaints the same thing). Especially since the incidence of thromboembolism (blood clots) in cancer patients is much higher than the general population at about fifteen percent. Luckily, all my tests came back okay and my heart rate improved after receiving two bags of IV fluids. The ER physician chalked it all up to dehydration. I am scheduled for another echo and I will see the cardio-oncologist this Thursday. I am curious to know if my heart function declined any further with the last round of chemo. Given my symptoms, it seems very possible. Fuck cancer!

November 4, 2019. After all the chest pounding and the whooshing in my head yesterday, I was afraid to go to sleep last night. I was afraid I wasn't going to wake up. I wrote a poem about it and then did a meditation. I feel a little better today—more fluttering than pounding. It is scary to feel this way! This is the first time I feel this way in the entire six months of my journey.

I will see the radiation oncologist this morning. The oncology social worker thinks I should stay off work until I'm completely done with treatment, but my oncologist will go along with anything I want to do (up to going back sixty percent max). Such tough decisions! Will I be able to handle all of it? My chemo brain has such difficulty with word finding still. And chemo fatigue is not anything you can just push through. It is feeling weak, a quick onset of tiredness that is not improved by sleep, sleeping all day, problems concentrating, heaviness in the muscles, and confusion. It is not your everyday should-have-slept-more fatigue. I also worry that doing osteopathic manipulation on patients will be exceedingly difficult because of the fatigue. And when I start radiation, I fear I will be uncomfortable from radiation burns and fatigue, and possibly from nausea due to the scatter. I also have to find a time to go to surgery to remove my right ovary and tubes. I need a magic wand to fix all of my symptoms and the psychic ability to know what my future looks like.

Still Here

She cannot sleep but she is so very tired.
Her Half functioning heart is deeply inspired.
She wants to write some words down just in case,
In case tonight is the night she goes to the place
Where she meets the angels or whatever comes after,
After a life well lived, full of tears and laughter.
She feels strange, like she is dying,
Weak, breathless, ears hear sighing.
Her chest has been pounding most of the day.
She goes to the hospital, they tell her she's okay.
She still feels strange and not quite right.
She looks in the mirror, the reflection of her light.
She is pale and bald and she looks so sick,
All she does is lie awake and watch the clock tick.
There is incredible fear tonight in going to sleep.
Will she wake up? The uncertainty makes her weep.
She has no thirst, isn't this a symptom of dying,
She wonders, she was once a doctor prying,
Prying for answers as she cared deeply for others.

The confident doctor now shrinks under the covers.
Wondering and waiting if tonight is the night,
Or if tomorrow will be better in the morning light.

November 6, 2019. I had a very vivid dream a couple of nights ago. In the dream, I was at a leadership conference for women physicians. It was similar to the real conference I went to at the Cleveland Clinic last September. In my dream, the conference was in Chicago and I remember all of the other women clicked together. I was the outcast. It was like Mean Girls had a conference. So I left the conference early and drove to my parents' house in Detroit. After arriving at my childhood home, one of my top front teeth fell out. When I awoke from this dream, I had a sinking feeling in my stomach that I was going to be fired for missing so much work. Today I talked with the HR manager and, although I am not being fired, they are allowed to post my position to make sure patients are taken care of. I will still be considered a hospital system employee on a medical leave of absence and I will maintain my benefits and health insurance. However, if they fill my position, I could be placed at another location. My dream now makes perfect sense—I feel like an outcast at work since I am on a leave of absence. And the tooth falling out has to do with my being confident to speak up for myself. I wish I could go back next week, but I am still so weak. Maybe it was a mistake to get the flu shot at my last chemo. Maybe my heart function has dropped some more. Maybe it's all in the universe's plan to lead me to what I am meant to do or become. Who knows what my future holds? Maybe I will be with UH or maybe some other entity. Only time will tell. But seriously, where is that goddamn crystal ball when you need it?

Chapter 41

"Courage is knowing it might hurt and doing it anyway. Stupidity is the same. And that is why life is hard!!!"—Jeremy Goldberg

November 8, 2019. Yesterday morning I had my fifth echo. It took forever to get all the images they needed and I had to get an IV image enhancer called Difinity. The echo went on for so long that it ran into my doctor's appointment with my cardio-oncologist. He came into the echo room while I was being scanned and he was able to determine that the ejection fraction was around forty-six percent. The good news is that my heart function has stabilized. The bad news is that forty-six percent is still below the normal range. My pre-chemo baseline was sixty to sixty-five percent. I have to keep taking my beta-blocker and getting monthly echoes. If my EF drops further, they will have to add another very specialized medication. They have to be careful what they give me because my blood pressure runs on the low side. Even when I satisfy my French-fry cravings, my blood pressure has been running 90-100 systolic. More good news is that I can continue my Herceptin infusions for now. That is a relief to me since I am told that Herceptin is a very important medication for my type of cancer. The cardiac symptoms I was having have improved. I can walk around my house without feeling short of breath and dizzy and as if I might pass out. There has been an improvement in the chest pounding, shortness of breath, and dizziness, whicht took me to the ER on Sunday with the fear of a blood clot in my lungs. It's the little things in life. I am not in heart failure, so my cardio-oncologist is attributing the symptoms to a cumulative side effect of all the chemotherapy I have had. He has not yet released me to return to work. I feel like a lab rat sometimes and I feel like I could make a full-time job with all of the appointments I have in the next couple of weeks. Next week I will have the first of two appointments for radiation planning.

In other news, my right ovarian mass and both fallopian tubes are scheduled to be removed on December 10. More body parts are being amputated. I feel like I am losing even more of my womanhood as time progresses. More grieving will take place. More fear. More uncertainty. More waiting for the pathology results wondering if this ovarian mass is benign or malignant.

As Elliot and I put up the Christmas tree tonight, I was pondering whether this Christmas would be my last. I am trying my best not to feed my fears, but they are there. The thoughts swirl through my mind like snow swirls through Cleveland. The snow isn't always there, even when it is cold. My fears aren't always at the forefront of my mind; they come and go like Cleveland snow.

November 10, 2019. Everyone has a different opinion about what courage is, but here's mine.

It is courageous to have some good days and not so good days and to be honest fowards yourself and your loved ones about it. It is courageous to be authentic and true to yourself. It is normal to ride the ups and downs of a serious medical issue and see the whole picture. It is extremely courageous to share your fears, share your vulnerability, and share ups and downs of your journey with others.

It is not courageous to have to constantly fake that everything is fine. It is not courageous if you have to "act tough" and never break down. It is not courageous (or normal) to be happy all the time. I will never be fake. Some days I will be happy and share good news. Some days I will be withdrawn and not want to talk. Some days I will be raging mad or crying my eyes out. And I will share it all. When you are going through difficult times or through something traumatic, all feelings are valid—anger, bewilderment, acceptance, joy, sadness, etc. And they demand to be felt.

November 13, 2019. There are two different kinds of radiation for treating cancer. The "standard of care" in treating breast cancer involves a photon beam (X-rays or gamma rays). The risks of radiation to the chest are skin dryness, itching, blistering or peeling, fatigue, lymphedema, and possible scarring to the surrounding organs. Since my cancer is on the left, there is potential damage to the heart, lung, or esophagus. If the lung is radiated, radiation pneumonitis (inflammation of the lung tissue) could result. There is more scatter with photons, and areas that shouldn't get radiated will be radiated. Proton beam is a newer technology. Protons do not penetrate as deeply and the stream is more precise. There is more risk of skin burns but less internal organ damage with protons. Proton beam is also triple the cost compared with photon beam. Today the radiation nurse called me stating my insurance will cover proton beam if I want to do it.

I suspect the reason they will cover proton beam is because my cancer is left-sided and I already have heart damage from chemotherapy. The other option is to contribute to science and enter the RADCOMP trial, which randomizes patients to either proton beam or photon beam radiation. The thought of contributing to science is a bit exciting. More so than the $400 the subjects in the trial get. I don't know what to do—proton or photon, or be put in a trial where either one is a fifty-fifty shot.

Tomorrow I will go in for my first of two staging visits before the radiation treatments actually start. I am scared of making the wrong decision. I don't want to do either. In addition, radiation can cause damage to the underlying ribs and soft tissues, leaving these areas prone to soft tissue tumors or rib fractures down the road. This seems like an important decision. I asked the radiation oncologist at my cancer center what would she do in this case and she simply said, "The trial."

I will get some more information tomorrow when I go for my staging visit. Maybe then the decision will be easier?

Chapter 42

"Be a lamp, a lifeboat, a ladder. Help someone's soul heal. Walk out of your house like a shepherd."—Rumi

November 15, 2019. Yesterday was my first of two radiation planning visits. The radiation oncology nurses took me to the radiation room. Then they put this stuff that reminded me of papier-mâché into a large blue plastic bag and had me lie on it to make a mold of my body. My radiation oncologist came in to talk with me and answer any questions I had. After they stuck stickers and marked up my body with green marker, they were ready to perform the scans. The radiation nurses told me I am not allowed to wash the marker off. It is bright green and rubbing off on my bra and clothes. I hope this green marker comes out of my clothes. I could not tell if they were using sharpies or Crayola.

Next step was a specialized CT scan. During the CT, I had to wear nose clips and put a mouthpiece in. I had been snorkeling in the Bahamas before and the device briefly reminded me of this time seven years ago when my best friend and I took a cruise and snorkeled with sea turtles in St. Thomas. I was quickly snapped back to reality when they told me to take a big breath and hold it for fifteen seconds. The radiation oncologist and the physicist will then look at plans for both proton and photon beam to see which looks like a better plan. I don't know enough information yet to make a decision but I certainly do not want to do any radiation that could damage my heart and lung. Everyone has a different anatomy so photon could be better than proton beam for some people. I will just have to wait and see. I already have heart damage from the Herceptin and Perjeta; I certainly don't want additional heart damage from radiation too. My cancer is/was left sided; too close to my half-functioning heart for comfort.

I feel incredibly lucky to be at a hospital that offers proton beam therapy. There are only two medical centers in the entire state of Ohio that offer it. University Hospitals in Cleveland and University of Cincinnati, Medical Center. I was a bit shocked when I found this out—I was surprised that Cleveland Clinic, the largest hospital system in Ohio, does not offer proton beam radiation. The radiation oncologist explained to me that, since UH has Rainbow, one of the biggest and best pediatric hospitals in the country, they possess a proton beam machine. Proton beam is more precise and they don't want little kids getting areas radiated that don't need to be. I told my radiation oncologist that I am still a kid. I feel like it some days in the cancer center that I am the youngest person there. On a serious note, I guess the universe has a way of working things out. I did my residency through Cleveland Clinic and then it did not work out for me to get an attending job within their health system when I was completing residency. I had offers from several places including Lake Health and University Hospitals. I have been with UH since 2010, almost ten years. As things come full circle as a physician, a donor, and a patient, I am so grateful for all of it.

Here is to bravely marching forward to the next leg of this ultra-marathon.

November 19, 2019. Let's start with the good news: my husband started a new job Friday as a substitute teacher's aide at our son's school. After being a stay-at-home parent for many years, a school ambassador, and frequent volunteer, it was a natural next step. I cannot wait to hear all the stories and the funny things the kids at Hawken Lower School (preschool and prekindergarten) say and do. When Elliot started preschool he was hilarious. For a while, he insisted his name was Buzz Lightyear.

Elliot celebrated grandparents' day with both sets of grandparents at his school today. No matter how hard that I try, I cannot picture what Elliot will be like as an adult. I wonder if he will give me grandkids. I am living one day at a time. I hope I will be alive in twenty years. Only time will tell. He is only in kindergarten, but Elliot has almost mastered the free style in swimming and is now going off the diving board. Not bad for a six-year-old.

Life is like a rollercoaster ride. This morning I puked so violently that I broke blood vessels below my eyes. I have no explanation, but perhaps it was due to sinus drainage or to taking zinc on an empty stomach? I took zinc and vitamin C hoping to avoid the lovely viruses kindergarteners like to bring home and share.

Today I went to my oncology appointment and found out that my blood counts are crazy low. My hemoglobin was only 5.2 (normal 12-16). It was such a low level that my oncologist and nurse came into the infusion suite while I was getting my Herceptin and Perjeta infusion. They were shocked that I was walking around that way, to say the least. They were in such disbelief that they sent in a phlebotomist to draw my blood from a peripheral vein. I have no veins; that's why I have a med port. I was a hard stick before cancer, but then chemo ruins your veins. She looked for veins everywhere, even my feet. She had to stick me twice (left hand and right wrist) to get blood. All of this nonsense just because the oncologist could not believe the lab result. The blood count was the same as the port draw. No wonder I have felt so weak and my heart has been pounding like crazy when I have tried to walk my dog. I am literally walking around with one third of my normal blood volume. Surprisingly, my vitals are stable at rest, so I am able to stay out of the hospital. (The oncologist doesn't want me catching anything else with my weakened immune system this time of year). I am shocked I am still upright with this low blood level. So I have to go into to the cancer hospital tomorrow for a blood transfusion. I don't know why I get these rare complications very few people get with my regimen. My bone marrow has taken a huge hit from this last chemo.

Okay, cancer, I am done with you and all of your complications!

Rollercoaster Ride

Here I was coasting through life
A woman, a doctor, a mother, a wife.
Then I am diagnosed with cancer in my breast.
Feels like getting on a rollercoaster being put to the test.
First I am deep down in the deepest tunnel,
My mind is swirling around like water in a funnel.
With much trepidation, I click my safety belt,
I get on the ride even though I want to just melt,
Melt into a puddle next to this scary ride.
There is no doubt in my mind, I just want to hide.
Surgery is over now, I am over the first big hill.
While healing at home, it seems like the ride is still.

Then out of nowhere, the rollercoaster takes a big drop,
There is cancer in my nodes, I want this ride to stop.
The next twist and turn of the ride is up ahead,
Chemotherapy is needed the oncologist said.
I endure five months of sickness, weakness and pain,
Anemia, heart damage, wear and tear of my brain.
When will the rollercoaster stop? How much more can I take?
I want to get off the ride, tell the operator to brake!
More twists, more drops, more tunnels so dark,
More surgery to remove yet another body part,
Then radiation treatments that could cause burns,
This is the scariest rollercoaster with all of its turns.
My life will never be the same after the ride ends,
But I can warn the person next in line what's around the bend.

November 20, 2019. I was supposed to get my blood transfusion at my regular outpatient chemo infusion clinic today at 11:00 am. That didn't happen. Somehow my blood type and screen didn't make it to the blood bank. Just as it is when traveling or wedding planning, not everything will go one hundred percent according to plan with cancer. Okay, no big deal, I went to the observation unit at the UH Seidman Cancer Center at the main campus. I got my blood drawn and then I had to wait two hours for the blood to come down from the blood bank. A very nice art therapist spent some time with me, helping me make two pieces of art. One was a collage of things that I was grateful for or made me happy. I put pictures of downtown Cleveland on it. Even though I was born and bred in Detroit, I do love Cleveland. I love the medical care. I love the restaurants. I love Playhouse Square, which is second to Broadway in the theater world. I love my friends here. The second piece of art I made was a painting. I painted an hourglass inside of an XO. It is a reminder to love thyself no matter how much or little sand there is inside the hourglass. My friend, another physician with cancer, came and sat with me and brought me a cake and drove me home from the hospital. More things to be grateful for.

I am extremely grateful for the blood donors, access to good care, and the nurses who cared for me, the art therapist, and my husband and friends.

My heart is full, literally and figuratively, since I just had a blood transfusion. Now my hands are a little pink after all the blood. My room in the cancer center had a big window and, just outside my window, there was a tree. It was barren of leaves and there was an empty nest. It reminded me that the leaves and the birds will return one day just like my hair and my health will come back. I think my hair is starting to grow. The follicles feel prickly and sensitive again, similarly to when my hair fell out. Also, there is some fuzz now on top of my head. When my head brushes against my pillowcase it feels like someone is rubbing sandpaper in certain spots on my scalp. Is this a good sign? One can hope!

Chapter 43

"Please grant me the serenity to stop beating myself up for not doing things perfectly, the courage to forgive myself because I always try my best, and the wisdom to know that I am a good person with a kind heart."—Eleanor Brownn

November 23, 2019. After being at the cancer center all day on Wednesday, I rested at home on Thursday. On Friday I went in to Connor Integrative for acupuncture, and the acupuncturist worked to stimulate my bone marrow, build blood, and help my hot flashes. The acupuncture must have helped because I felt better today. I am no longer hearing a whooshing sound in my head. Saturday was a good day overall, the peak of the rollercoaster instead of the valley. A friend invited me to an art gallery that was having an installment on social justice art. The pieces were all very moving. Saturday night my husband and I went out to dinner. Like the beautiful colors in a painting, the blood transfusion and the acupuncture came together perfectly in my body. I feel like, the moment I am able to move off the couch, I will seize the moment. There is an old saying that was inscribed on my high school, "When the sun shines, make hay." It's a piece of advice that has carried me through the years, even though I graduated from high school over twenty years ago. At this time in my life, the phrase translates to this: "Take advantage of your good days. You never know what tomorrow will bring."

November 27, 2019. I still don't have a start date for radiation but I did see the proton beam radiation oncologist (Dr. Harris) on Monday. I learned a lot. She said that there are really three types of radiation treatments available:

1. Whole beam radiation (fifty-nine-year-old photon technology).
2. IMRT (intensity modulated radiation therapy using photons).
3. Proton beam radiation.

She explained to me that everyone's anatomy is different and the plan needs to be individualized to the patient. For one patient, IMRT might be the best plan because of how it covers the area needing to be treated and spares the surrounding organs the best. For another patient, it may be equally beneficial to do proton therapy or IMRT. She wants me to choose the plan that gives me the lowest dose of radiation to my heart, which is already damaged from the chemo. I am still waiting to find out which plan this is. With cancer as my classroom, I just keep on learning.

In other news, I cancelled my surgery on December 10. Dr. Harris said it's not a good idea to have elective surgery in the middle of radiation treatments. I informed the gynecologic oncologist and she agreed. We will pick a date early next year to remove the tubes and right ovary.

I had acupuncture today and had my blood re-drawn. My blood counts are much better after the transfusion.
Hemoglobin is now 8.6 (normal 12-16).
White blood cells: 4.0 (normal 4-10).
Platelets: 160 (normal 150-400).

I am thankful for the good numbers. Hopefully my hemoglobin will continue to improve, and I will no longer need more blood transfusions. Thank you again to the two donors who gave blood; I don't know who you are. I do remember one unit was A- and the other was A+ and I didn't puke or have a transfusion reaction, so I am happy about that. Happy Thanksgiving!

December 2, 2019. Although Thanksgiving just ended, I am taking another moment to be thankful. As we head into the last month of 2019, I have to say that I am thankful for so many things.

I am thankful that my heart, although significantly weakened by my cancer treatments, is still pumping blood. I am thankful I can still walk, even when it's actually physically hard because I am anemic and have heart damage, and I am just plain wiped out from cancer treatments.

I am thankful when I have to tell myself that I will not die when my heart is pounding as if I was running into the wind up a steep hill. And when I get tired doing simple tasks, I am thankful for every ounce of breath in my lungs.

I am thankful for the ER doctors and nurses I have seen more than I ever planned to. And for not having to go to the ER or hospital this week (knock on wood!), I am thankful.

I am thankful for my husband, who has accompanied me to almost every doctor's appointment, test, and chemo treatment. I am thankful for handling all of the crazy ups and downs of this journey.

I am thankful for my oncology team who cares for me, listens to me, and calls to check on me. It means a great deal to me.

I am thankful for waking up every morning, especially after those nights I've fallen asleep unsure if I'll wake up the next day and then I open my eyes.

I am thankful for every single physician, nurse, medical assistant, technician, and receptionist who has seen me, really seen me as a person, for those who have been there for all the ups and downs, and for those who have offered snacks and blankets at chemo. I cannot thank them enough for listening to me.

I am thankful for those devastating tears threatening to drown me along the way, which have paved the way for gratitude and beautiful poetry. And for the realization that I am just a human being going through rough waters, I am thankful.

I am thankful for all of the incredible memories and for spending lots of time with my son. I've made these memories by *choosing* not to let cancer steal my joy, especially on days when I am feeling well.

I am thankful for those angels in my life who have not only showed up but have continually gone above and beyond in countless ways, you know who you are.

I am thankful for sweet doggy licks and snuggles when I needed them. I love you, Pooh Bear!

I am thankful for my physician cancer-sisters who are there for advice, virtual hugs and support, you are amazing!

I am thankful for my company that has given me the ability to take time off when I have needed it the most. And I am thankful for the insurance and the medical care provided by my system.

I am thankful for the journey over the past seven months that has been a rollercoaster ride, but that has paved the way for beautiful poetry and publications.

I am thankful for the discovery of coping mechanisms, for art therapy, for music therapy, for things I would have never delved into before, but have discovered their healing powers.

I am thankful for my life, the good parts, the bad parts, the hard parts, the hysterically funny parts and every minute in between.

I am thankful for it all.

Hope

Hope is feeling the fresh air and sun on my face.
Hope is waking up, being alive another day.
Hope is the strength to keep going, even if I am slow.
Hope is in that flower that shows me how to grow.
Hope is my neighbor bringing over treats.
Hope is the loved ones tending to my needs.
Hope is my doctors and nurses who help me get better.
Hope is the friends who send me cards and letters.
Hope is my dog who lets me snuggle his soft fur.
Hope is knowing how many things I've survived before.
Hope is sometimes elusive, at times in plain sight.
Hope is getting through cancer and being all right.
Hope is the strength to move forward up the hill.
Hope is mediating to find self-peace and be still.
Hope is knowing there are better days ahead.
Hope is smiling even when I feel like lead.
Hope is a dream of days without sadness and pain.
Hope is life without cancer and living again!

December 3, 2019. Today I had my sixth echo (heart ultrasound) and I made the technician tell me what the computer reading said. I needed a shred of good news today. The tech was sweet and she told me my ejection fraction even though they aren't really supposed to do that. The computer reading said my EF was forty-seven percent—stable and not significantly changed from last time. I am in that gray zone of not being well enough to exercise with my trainer at the gym, but not sick enough to qualify for cardiac rehab. I really wish that our hospital system had a cancer rehabilitation program. I am jealous that other hospitals have these programs, but our system doesn't. University of Vermont and University of North Carolina are two examples of hospitals that have these programs. I asked my cardio-oncologist, before he moved out of state around Thanksgiving, why UH does not have something like this. He told me it was because insurance companies don't want to cover it. He, too, thought it was a necessary program. The UNC program is funded by a grant and patients donate what they can—it could be $1 or $5 or whatever. Before I had cancer I would have never thought of this. But I am changed by this journey. I did a little digging and found out that both The Gathering Place and my local YMCA have cancer rehab programs. I am learning so many things I will be able to share with my patients. I am struck by the thought that I will never be the person I was before my cancer diagnosis.

I have a cardiology appointment coming up on Thursday and I am still waiting for my radiation schedule. Stay tuned.

December 6, 2019. When it rains, it pours! I am dealing with too much at once and feeling very irritable right now. First of all, my house is under construction. We had a shower built in the basement and it's leaking badly. When someone showers it produces a river of water flowing on the floor. And they already completely demolished the upstairs bathroom for a complete remodel. The Foreman and the plumber were able to identify the problem and they will be fixing it once the upstairs shower is done. Until then we are stuck with water all over the floor anytime someone showers. At least it's in the basement on the cement floor!

Secondly, I am so sick and tired of being asked every goddamn day when radiation starts. Everyone keeps asking. If I knew, I would have told you. I called the radiation oncology nurse yesterday and I *still* don't have a schedule. Come on people! I am feeling very antsy. I had my planning CT done almost a month ago (November 14) and I saw the radiation oncologist Monday to choose the plan (UH has two options: protons or photons). I chose one, so let's go people! Now, I am still waiting. I can't plan anything without this schedule and it is making my life a living hell. There is so much uncertainty in my life! Next person to ask me what I am doing for Christmas gets punched in the face. Hell, I don't know what I am doing tomorrow!

Lastly, I have been worrying for months about losing my job. When I missed my targeted return to work date because of fucking CANCER, the human resource manager told me that they could potentially fill my position since I have missed six months of work. Everyone I talked to kept reassuring me that I was crazy, that this would not happen. I heard things like, "Why would the system get rid of one of its best physicians for taking time off for cancer treatments." My gut instinct told me differently. This Monday I received an email from a hospital recruiter looking for a primary care physician for my old practice. As I have said before, my gut instinct rarely steers me wrong. I spoke with the HR manager and my medical director this afternoon. As it turns out, they *are* eliminating my position because "the system is trying to save money."

I checked the physician employee handbook and it does say they can terminate or fill your position after leave has exceeded twenty-six weeks (I'm at twenty-eight). I signed off in agreement to this handbook when I signed my contract. I am now in limbo. It's a scary place to be. It feels like I am falling without a net to catch me. Women in my support group said:

- "You will settle in and find where you belong."
- "It feels scary and uncertain but it might just be the beginning of a new (and better) chapter."
- "You have so many possibilities!"
- "Maybe this is the chance for youe to find a perfect opportunity that you wouldn't have looked for otherwise!"
- "Change can open new doors."

I know they are trying to be helpful but the "new doors will open" thing just sounds so clichéd. I cannot just leave and go to another health system. I cannot imagine leaving my current oncology team right in the middle of treatment. I am scared and stunned. I feel like I am being punished yet again for being sick. I even cancelled my ovary surgery so I could get back to work sooner. I want to get back to work, I really do! I am the one who pays the bills and carries the insurance for the family. I was just reflecting on how thankful I was for everything, but I am not thankful for this huge bump in the road. It's more than a bump; it's like skydiving when the parachute won't open. I am sure I will land on my feet...eventually. But right now, I am the one in chemopause with irritability and anxiety from all of these unknowns. And then, add on big hormone fluctuations.

As I am writing these words, tears prick at my eyes. Some people say that their cancer was a gift. Hell to the NO! Cancer is not a fucking gift. It is pain, surgeries, poison, radiation burns, and a zillion tests and doctor appointments. The treatment for the disease can cause more agony than the disease itself! Who knew? I sure as hell didn't.

Cancer patients endure so much. Medical appointments, biopsies, surgeries, pokes, blood draws, IV infusions, scans. Physically, there is pain, hair loss, nails crumbling, nausea, weakness, fatigue, diarrhea, constipation, cognitive changes, palpitations, dizziness, shortness of breath, metallic taste, and nerve damage. Emotionally, there is sadness, fear, anxiety, adjustment, grief, depression, agitation, frustration, bitterness, tension, feeling stunned, lost, desperate, trapped, helpless, hysterical, doubting exhausted, fragile, vulnerable, insecure, overwhelmed, motivated, eager, determined, inspired, loving, optimistic, thankful, grateful, and healed. And on top of all this, up to thirty percent of cancer patients experience job loss.

And this is just the tip of the iceberg.

The Sick Doctor

My son wrote this title, he was only five,
He knows his mom fights to stay alive.

Thirty-eight years old, a doctor and a mom,
Hit out of the blue by a ticking time bomb.

Doctors and mothers aren't supposed to get sick,
But here we are, the one cancer had to pick.

The sick doctor gets Surgery, Chemo, radiation, pills...
So many Tests and appointments—and what about the bills?

What about the trip we were supposed to take?
Missed out on Florida and wedding cake.

The sick doctor is home, too sick to work right now.
She worries about returning, mostly wondering how.

She worries about all of the questions the patients will have:
Where was my doctor? I waited day after day.

When will the sick doctor's life return to how it was?
When will she find that stride at work or on runs?

When will her eyebrows and hair grow back?
When will she get back her energy she lacks?

Only time and patience can heal this doctor's body and mind
No one has a crystal ball to give answers of that kind.

So she writes while she waits, one hour and day at a time,
She writes down her journey, she writes down her rhyme.

She spends time resting and, when she is feeling strong,
She goes outside for a walk and listens to Pink songs.

Her emotions will vary based on the day,
From fearful and anxious to strong and brave.

She longs for the day she will be free of the cancer chains,
Sometimes she smiles through the tear stains.

The sick doctor continues to bravely fight on,
Sharing her journey and all the ups and downs.

Bibliography

1. Emig, Mimi. "With a Little Help from My Friends." *Pulse-Voices from the Heart of Medicine.* Oct 6, 2019. https://pulsevoices.org/index.php/pulse-more-voices/more-voices-2019/how-can-i-help

2. Haefner, Megan. "Cancer forces 42% of patients to exhaust life savings in 2 years, study finds." *Becker's Hospital CFO Report.* October 4, 2018. https://www.beckershospitalreview.com/finance/cancer-forces-42-of-patients-to-exhaust-life-savings-in-2-years-study-finds.html

3. Lindberg, Eric. "Researchers uncover danger of ringing victory bell after cancer treatment." October 24, 2019.

4. Ritchie, Karen. MD "Angels and Bolters: A Field Guide to the Wildlife of Cancer." May 28, 2000. https://www.cancerlynx.com/angelsbolters.html

---

Suggested Reading:
1. Green, John. *The Fault in Our Stars.* New York, New York: Penguin, 2012.

2. Kalanithi, Paul. *When Breath Becomes Air.* First edition. New York: Random House, 2016.

3. Lucas, Geralyn. *Why I Wore Lipstick to my Mastectomy.* New York: St. Martin's Press, 2004.

Acknowledgements

I would like to thank everyone who helped me get through the roughest 7 months of my entire life. Thank you to my husband, Marty, who showed up every day for this. And to my son, Elliot, who came up with the idea of writing this book. Thank you to Anne Trubek at Belt Publishing for helping my book become a reality. A special thanks to Dr. Lisa Rock for being a rockstar surgeon. To all the awesome people at Seidman Cancer center. To Allecia and Mercedes for listening to me vent. To Dr. Paula Silverman and Rachel, my medical oncology team, for putting up with me at my worst. To my chemo nurses, especially Jen, for your compassion. To Dr. Janice Lyons, Liz, David, and Micky, my radiation team, for being so respectful and gracious. To Eileen, for always knowing the right thing to say. To my parents, family, and friends who stuck by me-you know who you are-thank you from the bottom of my heart for all of the encouragement!

www.ingramcontent.com/pod-product-compliance
Lightning Source LLC
Chambersburg PA
CBHW051738020426
42333CB00014B/1369